Disability Pension

Disability Pension:

A Treaty in Insurance Medicine

Edited by

Ioana Soare

Cambridge Scholars Publishing

Disability Pension: A Treaty in Insurance Medicine

Edited by Ioana Soare

This book first published 2025

Cambridge Scholars Publishing

Lady Stephenson Library, Newcastle upon Tyne, NE6 2PA, UK

British Library Cataloguing in Publication Data
A catalogue record for this book is available from the British Library

ISBN: 978-1-0364-4801-1
ISBN (Ebook): 978-1-0364-4802-8

To my supportive family,

Viorel, Mina and Oana

TABLE OF CONTENTS

Part 9 Ethics

FOREWORD

This treaty is the result of an effort to understand and explain the concepts in the field of the insurance medicine, especially the social medicine.

A big Thank you to all my colleagues from EUMASS, ICLAM and the Romanian societies of medical expertise, who have helped along this journey.

Mostly I want to thank the publishing team from Cambridge Scholars Publishing, who have encouraged and helped me to produce this book, a tool that I hope will be useful to all those who want to learn and practice in this domain.

—Ioana Soare

INTRODUCTION

The insurance medicine allows a complete assessment of the patient, both now and as risks in the future, based on the statistical tables. These statistical limits of the body's structural or functional parameters, as well as the data obtained through the evidence-based medicine, were identified in the Caucasian (especially Anglo-Saxon) populations and led to the standardization of the patient assessment (e.g. the tables for spirometry, ECG, EEG, BMI, the risk calculation tables in the arterial hypertension or the diabetes, etc..).

In medicine, today, we know what the future holds. We can say with 70-80% accuracy, what life span we expect a person to have and what disease predispositions they have, based on the life expectancy calculated in the respective population and the risks of having certain conditions, personal risks (genetic, related to eating habits or sports), risks related to the profession and others.

How much the science has evolved! NO. These things were known from the year 1700, if not from the year 1600, by the Anglo-Saxon populations, based on the town halls civil status registers.

The insurance, in various forms, is very old and relates to a tendency towards stability, security and lack of worry about tomorrow, natural desires. The first documented attestations date back to the time of the Egyptians, Phoenicians and the Chinese, who also had a form of insurance in trade. Romans also had the notion of pension, annuity.

At first only the healthy people were insured. The insurance for individuals with various conditions only became possible in 1919, through the use of a substandard risk classification system.

In the last 40 years medicine has begun to take these notions into account, and thus the classifications and the risk stratifications for high blood pressure and diabetes have emerged. Only so the study of the **evolution** and **prognosis** of the diseases, the avoidance of the events (for example vascular accidents, some complications), the **extension of the life span** and above all the addition of quality-adjusted life year (QALY) were of greater importance, compared to the treatment of the diseases only. DALY, Disability Adjusted Life Years is an important statistical tool also. The

Evidence Based Medicine EBM appeared because of the need in insurance medicine to quantify, to precisely evaluate the functional deficit of the patient.

All these elements have moved from the statistics to medicine, because of the insurance companies. The money dictated order.

The disability assessment is the biggest and most challenging part of the insurance medical expert's activity.

This treaty will tackle the difficult aspects of the definitions, a comparison of criteria for patient evaluation, some aspects of the risks, the evolution and the prognosis.

The Chapter Brain Tumors Presumed Malignant Without Biopsy - Evaluation and Treatment Problems, was first published in a reduced form as an article in Austin Journal of Clinical Neurology, Volume 8 Issue 2-2021. The Chapter Rehabilitation for visually impaired people was first presented at the Conference: Family Medicine, the Cornerstone of Modern Medicine, 15th Edition, Volume of summaries, September 5-7, 2024, Etna Medical Publishing House, ISBN 978-630-6644-03-2.

In separate chapters, we discuss the disability from accidents (both work and road accidents) and the work-related diseases.

In the last chapter we debate the ethics. Is it ethical to hire an insurance medical expert in an insurance company? Can or may the hired physicians represent the best interesses of the patient? Should the medical expert be independent?

—Ioana Soare

PART 1

GENERAL INFORMATION

CHAPTER 1

NOTIONS USED IN INSURANCE MEDICINE

IOANA SOARE

Insurance is a means of protection against the financial loss [1]. An entity that provides insurance is known as an insurer, insurance company, or insurance carrier. A person or entity that buys insurance policies is known as an insured [1].

The insurance transaction involves: the insured assumes a relatively small guaranteed loss, known as a payment to the insurer, in exchange for the insurer's promise to compensate the insured in the event of a loss. The loss may not be financial in nature, but must be reducible to a financial point of view and must involve something in which the insured has an established insurable interest - property, possession or a pre-existing relationship [1].

The insured receives a contract, called an insurance policy, which details the terms and circumstances under which the insured will be financially compensated. The amount of money charged by the insurer from the insured, for the coverage set out in the insurance policy, is called premium (noun with psychological connotation) and is actually a rate payable periodically from the contract value. If the insured suffers a loss that is potentially covered by the insurance policy, the insured submits a claim to the insurer.

Social security - represents a social insurance program, supported by the state, which provides social protection against the factors that affect the well-being and the economic security of the population - poverty, old age, disability, lack of a job, etc... [2].

The social security provides basic coverage for the risks "sickness/ maternity/disability/death", "work accidents/occupational diseases", "old age" and "family". They cover different areas: the general regime, the agricultural regime and other special regimes. This also includes the social assistance, which supports the most disadvantaged.

The social insurance/social benefits are based on the principle of solidarity and contribution (in Romania, France, Germany - not in the UK, where the benefits are fixed amounts). All citizens have the same rights (the contracts are identical, not negotiable), binding on the territory of a country and guaranteed by the state. This includes the **medical leave** (short term sick leave), the **disability pension or benefit** (the long-term sick leave), the **survivor's pension**, the allowances and benefits for people with special needs (handicap), as well as others that are not the subject of the insurance medicine - the unemployment benefit, the death benefit, etc... [2,3]. To be detailed in the next chapter.

Adaptive incapacity/disability - represents the reduction of the possibility to perform a motor or cognitive activity, under conditions considered normal, due to the inherited or acquired deficiencies [2]. Can be defined also as any impairment that limits a person's ability to perform a certain activity (activity limitation) or interact with the environment (participation restriction). Two people with the same type of disability can be affected in very different ways [2,4].

Annuity - the companies that sell us annuities are betting on our lives - they are gambling. The annuities appeared in Roman times and were used by the town halls or kingdoms (England, Holland) to collect money.

The individual pays a fixed amount, for a number of years, and then receives regular payments for the rest of his live. If he dies before a company has paid the full value of the purchase price, the company makes a profit. If the individual lives longer, the company loses. The company averages all buyers and its profit is regulated by law to prevent abuse.

Edmund Halley made a study of the registers of the city of Breslau around the year 1700. He calculated the annual rate of deaths and births, drew up tables like Graunt's, used to calculate the annuities and the life insurance amounts. Consequently, the predictions could be made about the future by calculating the age at which a man might die [1].

Deficiency - the functional deficit - represents any disruption of the body's structure and/or of the normal physical or mental functions [4].

Disease - represents the organic or functional modification of the body's normal balance; the pathological process affecting the body; the illness, sickness, affection; the disturbance of the normal state of an organism [4].

Disability is a generic negative term for the impairments, activity limitations and participation restrictions. It denotes the contextual factors (environmental and personal factors) [2,3,4].

Disability- The Merriam Webster Dictionary proposes the following definition: the temporary or permanent state of being unable to work due to illness or injuries. The Cambridge Dictionary proposes: the condition of being unable to work because of health problems, and receiving money from a government or organization because of this. To be detailed in the next chapter.

Doctrine of chances by Reverend Bayes. How can we use the probabilities to measure the probability of not being wrong, when trying to predict a particular event? His method can guide us when our intuition is wrong. For example, suppose you are testing for a rare cancer with an incidence of 1% in the population. The test comes out positive. The test gives 21% false positive results. How likely are you to have cancer? Most people would answer that if the reliability of the test is 80%, then that is the probability. Using Bayes' formula, the correct probability is only 5% [1].

Gaussian curve, of the normal distribution of the random observations, is the basis for estimating the value of the data. The business people use it to plan the business development, the politicians to determine policies, the teachers to grade the students, the pollsters to analyze their data and make predictions, the medical researchers to test the effectiveness of various treatments, the economists to analyze the economic performance, the biologists to study the plant growth, the psychologists to analyze the human behavior, and the insurance companies to set their insurance premiums [1].

Handicap - represents a social disadvantage, resulting from a physical, mental or sensory deficiency, which affects and limits the persons normal social role, in accordance with age, sex, its environment [4].

Health - is defined by WHO as a state or feeling of well-being from a physical, mental and social point of view, not just the absence of disease. May be defined as a state of an organism untouched by any disease, in which the functioning of all organs is normal.

Invalidity - Invalid means not valid/ not normal, not a whole, bodily infirm. This word was used since the wars, especially the First World War, mainly for the soldiers returning home without some bodily parts. Represents also a person enfeebled by illness or injury [4].

In some countries, invalidity matches disability, but some consider an invalid as a person with disabilities, who is retired (long-term sick leave), as in Romania.

Life expectancy - John Graunt, born in 1620 in London made a study: Natural and political observations based on the obituaries - concerning the fertility, health, diseases, longevity, the ratio of sexes and the ages of mankind. Based on this statistical study, he published the Statistical Table of Life Expectancy, the basis of the life insurance industry, of the medical statistics and the demographic, the government statistics (the political arithmetic). The Dutchman Christiaan Huygens introduced the notion of Hope (hopeful gain) [1].

Life expectancy: The insurance companies look at it as a bet on the customer's lifetime (guesstimation). It is estimated a posteriori, because the probability values corresponding to various events have been determined by the objective process of counting outcomes in real-world experiences [10].

The Bernoulli family of mathematicians from Basel, Switzerland were involved in the probability theory. In 1713, the idea that a man could plan his life in a rational way, that minimized risk and maximized opportunity, was widely accepted. It was and it is done based on how to calculate the probabilities of the future events. Graunt's life expectancy tables and N. Bernoulli's use of probabilities in courts of law provided a numerical measure of a person's confidence in knowing a particular event [1].

The utility measures the significance of a particular outcome to a particular individual. It is a subjective notion, compared to the notion of hope, which is a mathematical notion.

Life insurance - represents a type of insurance through which the insurer pays a sum of money after a preset period or upon the death of the insured person [6].

Long-term care insurance - the insurance that refers to the payment of a monthly amount, in the event of the need for care over 60 days, for patients who cannot serve themselves. It represents a variety of social and health services provided for a period ongoing or extended, to people who need assistance, due to mental or physical disabilities [6].

The patient's circuit is the path taken by him from the moment of the first consultation with the doctor, for the purpose of diagnosis, his orientation towards medical, social and educational services, until the completion of the treatment and his integration into the community. For example, in rare diseases, we have an average of 7 YEARS until diagnosis, although in more than 50% of cases, the motor or sensory changes appear in the adulthood - the patients actively participate and are interested in solving their problem.

Quality of life (QoL) - holistic concept in order to be able to quantify and analyze the 4 dimensions of the health status:

- the physical condition and performance;
- the psychological well-being (self-esteem, cognitive performance, interpersonal relationships);
- the positioning and social relations;
- the economic status.

The quality of life - in the sense of the WHO definition, means the perception of individuals on their social situations, depending on their own needs.

Recovery - is a complex field of activity, medical, educational, social and professional, which aims to restore as fully as possible the functional capacity, lost or undeveloped by an individual, following an illness or trauma, as well as the development of the compensatory mechanisms to ensure, in the future, the possibility of working or self-serving, respectively an independent life from an economic and/or social point of view (WHO definition) [4].

The recovery plan - implies a multidisciplinary team; provides periodic evaluations for the reanalyze of therapeutic needs, according to the age; supports the patient throughout his life; it is mandatory by law (eg Law 360/2023 in Romania) for patients who receive social insurance rights. It contains medical actions, professional actions (reduced schedule, job adaptation, retraining) and social actions (discussions with the family, etc.) [4].

Return to work - RTW, established expression, which refers to the return to work of an employee, who was ill - the rehabilitation/ recovery of the work capacity [5].

Special educational requirements - the specific requirements or needs regarding the education, for the equalization of opportunities in the school and the social integration. These requirements are the consequences of a functional deficit, of some poor psycho-affective, socio-economic or life conditions, placing the individual in a state of difficulty in relation to his peers, not allowing him to make the most of his intellectual and aptitude potential, inducing a feeling of inferiority.

Work capacity - expresses a relationship between the morphological and functional potential, and the demands of the work, on the other hand [4].

References

1. Keith Devlin, The unfinished game, Humanitas, 2015, p 121, 131, 135
2. https://www.cdc.gov/ncbddd/disabilityandhealth/disability.html
3. Claudia Marinache, Disability Neuroscience, 2009, p 175-177
4. Şirjiţă Nicolae, &all, Elements of medical expertise and recovery of work capacity, Tiparg, 2014, p 14
5. (A guide to) Non-contributory Benefits for Disabled People and their Caretakers, Department for Work and Pensions, 2003, Belmont Press
6. https://en.wikipedia.org/wiki/Life_insurance

CHAPTER 2

DISABILITY

IOANA SOARE

The people with disabilities represent a major political and social objective all over the world. This disadvantaged category needs protection and integration into the society by implementing an improved legislative framework for the social insurance system [1].

The disability insurance or the life insurance policies provide an income replacement, when the insured is disabled because of accident or sickness.

The WHO defines it as follows: "Disabilities is an umbrella term. The disability is reflecting an interaction between the characteristics of a person's body and the particular features of the society, in which the individual lives" [2].

Disability - Limitation in people's activity due to health conditions, for at least the past 6 months [EU].

Some consider the disability tied to the work capacity.

The USA Social Security Administration defines the disability in terms of inability to perform a substantial gainful activity (SGA), by which it means "work paying minimum wage or better". The agency pairs SGA with a "listing" of medical conditions that qualify individuals for the benefits.

Disability can be defined in the insurance contracts in a number of different ways. These are:

- The inability of the insured to perform the duties of his or her occupation,
- The inability of the insured to perform the duties of any occupation for which he or she is fit, on the basis of experience, education, or training and

- The inability of the insured to perform any kind of work [3,5].

The disabled people require some protection measures in support of the social recovery and integration [5].

A kind of "people first" terminology is also used in the UK, but more often in the form "people with impairments". However, in the UK, the term "disabled people" is generally preferred to "people with disabilities". It is argued under the social model, that while someone's impairment (e.g. having a cataract) is an individual property, "disability" is something created by external societal factors, such as a lack of wheelchair access to their workplace. The term "disabled people" as a political construction is also widely used by international organizations, such as Disabled Peoples' International (DPI) [3].

Two conceptual models are more important in understanding the disability:

The medical model of disability

This model presents the disability as a problem of the person, directly caused by some health conditions. In the medical model, the management of the disability is aimed at a "cure", by the individual's adjustment and the behavioral change. For this type of perceiving disability, the principal response at the political level is that of reforming the healthcare policy [1,4].

The social model of disability

The issue of "disability" is seen as a socially created problem and a problem of the full integration of individuals into the society (see Inclusion (disability rights)). In this model, the disability is not an attribute of an individual, but rather a complex collection of conditions, many of which are created by the social environment. Hence, the management of the problem requires social action and is the collective responsibility of the society at large, to make the environmental modifications necessary for the full participation of the people with disabilities in all areas of the social life. The issue is both cultural and ideological, requiring an individual, community and a large-scale social change. From this perspective, the equal access for someone with an impairment/ disability is a human rights issue of major concern [3].

People can acquire disabilities at any point in their lives. Of critical importance is the ability to develop or maintain a high quality of life after the acquisition of a disability [3].

Conclusions

The term disability includes the imbalances, the limitations, the restrictions of the patients in their daily life.

Each country applies its national criteria under their legislation, when to decide the degree of disability, thus including or excluding people in this category, for political reasons.

Many insurance companies have also some lists of possible diseases, which quality for the disability benefits.

References

1. Mirica, Roxana & Soare, Ioana. (2020). The Evolution of Disability during the Last Years in Romania and EU Member States. Open Journal of Preventive Medicine. 10. 169-174. 10.4236/ojpm.2020.107012.
2. https://www.afro.who.int/health-topics/disabilities
3. Marshall Wilson Reavis III, Insurance: Concepts &Coverage, 2012, FriesenPress, p 85, 88
4. Committee on the Rights of Persons with Disabilities – 10 May 2017, CRPD/C/IRN/CO/1, para.8(a)
5. Anghelescu Aurelian, Bușcă Mihai, Constantin Adina, Andone Ioana, Anghelescu Lucia Ana-Maria, Onose Gelu – Employment of People with Disabilities in Romania. International Archives of Medicine. Section: Global Health and Health Policy.2016, vol 9 (365).

PART 2

EXPLAINING PENSIONS

CHAPTER 1

HISTORY

IOANA SOARE

Social security represents the state assistance to those lacking in economic security and welfare, e.g. the aged and the unemployed.

- **social insurance**, where people receive benefits or services in recognition of contributions to an insurance scheme. These services typically include the provision for retirement pensions, the disability insurance, the survivor benefits and the unemployment insurance.
- **income maintenance**—mainly the distribution of cash in the event of interruption of the employment, including the retirement, the disability and the unemployment.
- **services** provided by the administrations responsible for the social security. In different countries this may include the medical care, the aspects of social work and even the industrial relations.

More rarely, the term is also used to refer to **basic security**, a term roughly equivalent to access to basic necessities—things such as food, clothing, shelter, education, money, and medical care [1].

Social security is primarily a social insurance program providing social protection. Social security may refer to recognized conditions, including poverty, old age, disability, unemployment and others.

- **700 BCE** - The first insurance funds, in close connection with the maritime trade - Rhodes - some groups of merchants whose goods were part of a common transport, paid a sum of money, which was collected in a common fund, and this was used in case the goods of one of them was damaged or lost during the voyage [2].
- **600 BCE** - The first life insurances appeared in Ancient Greece and Rome. The tradesmen's guilds, called "benevolent societies", initiated common funds, used when one of the members died, with the aim of supporting his family.

- **1310** AD, the Duke of Flanders decided to establish the Insurance Chamber in Bruges for insurance against the maritime risks.
- **1601**, in London, the Parliament developed the regulations regarding this activity, by issuing the "Law on insurance policies used between traders" [2].
- 1688 - one of the first insurance companies in the world, Lloyd's was founded in England. The first life insurances were made for sailors.
- 1830 -In Romania, the first sickness pensions were granted for the wounded soldiers, the war invalids. They obtained the first invalidity pensions, which were regulated by the Organic Regulation, just like in Russia and Germany, France. Then the civil servants, miners, and after 1900 other categories of workers received social protection [3].
- **1883** - Germany enacted a compulsory sickness insurance law [1].
- **1889** - Germany enacted the compulsory old age insurance -which included the invalidity insurance - **the Bismarck law**, the first official pyramidal system financed by a tax on workers [4]. The other countries followed, maintaining this system till today. Because of the ageing population, the pyramidal scheme is very difficult to sustain. Unlike the Accident Insurance and the Health Insurance programs, this program covered from the start Industrial, Agrarian, Artisans and Servants. The Disability Insurance program was intended to be used by those permanently disabled [3,4].

References

1. www.socialsecurity.gov
2. Callund, David F. Pensions in Russia 2001, www.callund.com/pensionsrussia.pdf
3. www.wikipedia.com
4. https://socialwelfare.library.vcu.edu/social-security/social-security-a-brief-history-of-social-insurance/

CHAPTER 2

PENSIONS

IOANA SOARE

Europe had to wait for more than 100 years to modify this system. In the last 30 years, the European Union was born and has developed its structures. The language and the legislation needed harmonization, not the least in the field of the insurances. In 1987 - Geneva Association for the Study of Insurance Economics launched a research program called The Four Pillars" [1].

- First Pillar - the "State" pension, with mandatory contribution as a percentage of the salary, is based on a Bismarck-type pyramid system, without accumulation, interest, and is guaranteed by the state. The funds accumulated this month are consumed next month. The rulers of Europe did not know how to abandon this outdated system and make the transition to something else. That is why they introduced pillar 2, 3 and 4 in the EU [2].
- The Second Pillar - the mandatory private pension - Mandatory pension, withheld from salary, with both state and private managed funds. At the legal retirement age, the individual will receive a monthly amount, calculated on the basis of his contributions and the contract concluded with an insurance company, a standard contract, non-negotiable [2].
- Third Pillar - the private pension - Optional, private pension - the individual can join any private pension fund, which will manage the money independently. At the legal retirement age, the individual will receive either a monthly amount, calculated by the insurance company and included in the contract, or a total amount, included in the contract, which represents the initially agreed amount plus interest and the return on the investment made by the insurer. These funds are exclusively privately managed, but both the employee and the employer benefit from tax deductions. The disability and death clauses are included [2].

- 4th Pillar - optional, private pension and life insurance - It is actually a private life insurance with a pension component. The life insurance has a health insurance component (covers the sick leave, hospitalizations, accident disability pension, death) and a pension component managed by an investment fund. At the legal retirement age, the individual will receive either a monthly amount, calculated by the insurance company and included in the contract, or a total amount, included in the contract, which represents the initially agreed amount plus interest and the return on the investment made by the insurer. The health insurance part is not cumulative - it is money that the individual gives each year and does not get back - as with state health insurance [2].

The Treaty from Lisbon established in 2009 the steps to improve the social protection in Europe, considering the next 50 years, with scarce working force and a lot of old citizens.

The Treaty of Lisbon (initially known as the Reform Treaty) is an international agreement, that amends the two treaties which comprise the constitutional basis of the European Union (EU). The Lisbon Treaty amended the Treaty on the European Union (more commonly known as the Maastricht Treaty) and the Treaty establishing the European Community (the Treaty of Rome), renamed to the Treaty on the Functioning of the European Union (TFEU).

The three-pillar system consisting of a national defined contribution scheme (NDC contributory pension scheme), a capitalized pension scheme supported by state and private pension schemes, was the solution at hand [4].

Funds

Many countries have created funds for their citizens and residents to provide income when they retire (or in some cases become disabled). Typically this requires payments throughout the citizen's working life in order to qualify for benefits later on. A basic state pension is a "contribution based" benefit, and depends on an individual's contribution history [5].

In an unfunded defined benefit pension scheme, no assets are set aside and the benefits are paid for by the employer or other pension sponsor. The pension arrangements provided by the state in most countries in the world are unfunded, with the benefits paid directly from the current workers' contributions and taxes. This method of financing is known as Pay-as-you-go (PAYGO or PAYG). The social security system in the USA and most European countries are unfunded, having benefits paid directly out of the current taxes and social security contributions, while in Canada the wage-based retirement plan (CPP) is funded, with the assets managed by the CPP Investment Board. In some countries, such as Germany, Austria and Sweden, the companies run the retirement plans, often unfunded.

In a funded plan, the contributions from the employer, and sometimes also from the plan members, are invested in a fund towards meeting the benefits. The future returns on the investments, and the future benefits to be paid, are not known in advance, so there is no guarantee that a given level of contributions will be enough to meet the benefits. Typically, the contributions to be paid are regularly reviewed in a valuation of the plan's assets and liabilities, carried out by an actuary, to ensure that the pension fund will meet future payment obligations. This means that in a defined benefit pension, the investment risk and the investment rewards are typically assumed by the sponsor/employer and not by the individual [2].

The legislation for the social protection in the world is parted into:

- type A legislation, in which you are protected independently of how long you have worked or how much you have earned;
- type B legislation, in which you are protected accordingly to how much you have contributed (the Bismarck scheme, practically a pyramidal system).

It is much easier in the private insurance field - you are protected accordingly to how much you have contributed.

The type A legislation we can find in the UK, Denmark and the Netherlands - the flat-rate state pension, plus additional pension [5].

The type B legislation we can find in Romania, Austria, Germany, Latvia, Lithuania, Slovakia, Russia [2,4,5].

Many states, not only in Europe, have considered very difficult to sustain such schemes alone, because of the aging tendency of the population.

In Australia

The Age pension was the first payment issued from the Commonwealth Government and dates back to 1909. It is available to men aged 65 years and over. The age for women to become eligible is being progressively phased upward from 60 to 65 years, in line with the men.

Unlike the pension payments of many other countries, the **workers do not contribute to a pension or an insurance within Australia, and the payment is available after means testing.** This ensures that only those that require assistance receive it.

In Australia, most benefits are subject to a means test, a determination of whether an individual or family is eligible for help from the government. This will be done so according to the income.

Means-testing has been criticized. For example, William Beveridge, in the Beveridge Report (blueprint for the UK's post-war social system) was opposed to means-testing, due to the poverty trap (below). The difficulties of a poverty program versus a social program include:

Stigma - A program benefiting only the poor may carry a stigma on its use, and be demeaning.

Political support - A program benefiting only the poor may lack broad-based political support, in contrast to the programs that all share in.

Redistribution - The poverty programs transfer money from the rich to the poor, as they benefit the poor only, but are paid for by all.

Poverty trap - Means tests, particularly sharp cut-offs, create high marginal tax rates and can serve to keep people in poverty, both by removing the social support as the person tries to escape poverty, and by discouraging such attempts by the high costs. For example, the asset-based limits, such as requiring an individual to have little or no savings to qualify, not only discourage the saving (because of the cost of being disqualified from such savings) but require a person to become completely destitute to qualify, thus meaning that they do not have any much-needed savings when attempting to escape poverty.

Access - Means tests complicate the access to programs – many individuals who qualify for the programs, may not benefit from them.

Administrative costs - Means tests increase the administrative costs due to the verifications.

Entitlement/promises - If means-testing is implemented in an existing program, particularly for which people have paid taxes but not benefited, as in pensions or medical insurance, the reduction in benefits can be seen as a breach of promise and entitlement of the program [2, 3].

Conclusion

The similarities between the social insurance programs and the private insurance programs considering pensions, include:

- Wide pooling of risks;
- Specific definitions of the benefits provided;
- Specific definitions of the eligibility rules and the amount of coverage provided;
- Specific premium, contribution or tax rates required to meet the expected costs of the system.

The differences between the private and the social insurance programs include:

Equity versus Adequacy: The private insurance programs are generally designed with accent on the equity between the individual purchasers of coverage, while the social insurance programs generally emphasize the social adequacy of the benefits for everybody.

Voluntary versus Mandatory Participation: The participation in the private insurance programs is often voluntary, and where the purchase of insurance is mandatory, individuals usually have a choice of insurers. The participation in the social insurance programs is generally mandatory, and where the participation is voluntary, the cost is subsidized to ensure the universal participation.

Contractual versus Statutory Rights: The right to benefits in a private insurance program is contractual, based on an insurance contract. The insurer generally does not have an unilateral right to change or terminate the coverage before the end of the contract period (except in such cases as non-payment of premiums). The social insurance programs are not generally based on a contract, but rather on a statute, and the right to benefits is thus statutory, rather than contractual. The provisions of the program can be changed, if the statute is modified.

Funding: The individually purchased private insurance generally must be fully funded. The full funding is a desirable goal for the private pension plans as well, but is often not achieved. The social insurance programs are often not fully funded.

The rules on the social security coordination do not replace the national systems with a single European one. All countries are free to decide who is to be insured under their legislation, which benefits are granted and under what conditions. The EU provides common rules to protect the social security rights when moving within Europe (EU 27 + Iceland, Liechtenstein, Norway and Switzerland).

Some of the benefits/insurance rights are exportable in EU, considering that the expression "…….. resident" became "EU resident". See the Hendrix case [6].

References

1. https://en.wikipedia.org/wiki/Four_Pillars_(Geneva_ Association)
2. www.wikipedia.com
3. www.socialsecurity.gov
4. www.mmuncii.ro
5. www.eumass.com
6. www.eucaselaw.info/hendrix-2007/

CHAPTER 3

INTERNATIONAL DISABILITY PENSIONS

IOANA SOARE

In the European Union, the patient must apply for long term sick leave/ disability pension in the country where he contributed to the pension fund. There he is assessed by an insurance physician, according to the legislation of the respective country, and there he will receive the invalidity or old age pension [1].

There are patients who live in another state than the one where they worked. In the European Union, they must apply for the disability pension where they live, ask for a medical evaluation according to the E213/S1 form, which will be completed by a physician chosen by the local pension house. Then the form will be officially sent to the pension house in the country where the individual was employed. There the form will be examined, together with other medical documents, by another expert physician, who will grant the insurance rights according to the legislation of the paying country, which differs most of the time [1].

The time period worked in another EU country is recognized as length of service in Romania, but is paid only in the country where the individual contributed. There are other states implied in such treaties:

- Armenia
- Belarus
- Canada
- Ukraine
- Macedonia,
- The Kingdom of Morocco
- The Republic of Moldova,
- The UK
- The Russian Federation
- Turkey,

- The South Korea,
- Israel [2].

References

1. Soare Ioana, International Pensions - Insurance Medicine, Etna Publishing House, 2010
2. www.cnpp.ro

PART 3

INSURANCE MEDICINE

CHAPTER 1

MEDICAL EXPERTISE - SOCIAL AND PRIVATE INSURANCE MEDICINE

IOANA SOARE

Medical expertise, named also **social medicine, insurance medicine**, legal and insurance medicine, expert medicine is the clinical medical specialty, which **deals with the patient assessment, risk assessment**, functional deficit assessment (adaptive disability expressed as a percent) and the recovery and reintegration measures of the patient in the social and professional life, **in order to obtain some insurance rights** [1].

The notion of expertise designates a means of proof, representing the finding or opinion of a specialist in a specific field of knowledge, for the purpose of clarifying the factual matters. **The expertise is considered a scientific assessment of evidence** [2].

This specialty is called insurance medicine (Netherlands, Belgium, USA). In some countries it is considered a specialization within the legal medicine - Italy, Spain, Portugal, being called Legal and insurance medicine. In Germany, there is a separation between the social medicine and the insurance medicine [1]. In Romania it is defined as medical expertise.

ASIM/ Swiss definition: The insurance medicine deals with medical issues that are important for the development and implementation of public, social security or private insurance models. The insurance medicine is a medical specialty, which must include knowledge from all the major medical fields and the specialized clinical disciplines [3].

AIM Japan: The insurance medicine is an applied science built on the prognosis studies on the human disease and human longevity, integrating various disciplines required for the sound management of the life insurance business, including law, economics, sociology and mathematics, as well as the basic and clinical medicine [4].

The industry is recognized by the American Medical Academy, where the AAIM holds a seat [5].

The insurance medicine is a challenging and rewarding discipline.

It deals with the assessment of the health problems concerning the insurance claims, the effectiveness of interventions in terms of prevention, integration and reintegration, the insurance-related changes in the health of the population and the organization for the insurance solutions from a medical point of view. In the clinical practice, it also deals with the relationships between the patients, the insurance companies and the medical providers for appropriate medical services [3].

Why should the patient be examined?

1. Because he can declare the diseases he does not have.

2. Because he can hide the diseases he has.

3. Because he may have diseases he doesn't know he has.

Why was the medical expertise needed?

From ancient times, the medical and religious activities merged, because they were not understood and explained. They were fulfilled by the shaman. He did not lead the tribe. The head of the tribe had the capacity to control the shaman, to punish him.

In the Code of Hammurabi we have also recorded punishments applied to the doctors.

Why do people try and try again to question, to verify - because they don't understand, it's not explained to them and especially because they have the hope of healing.

We must also talk about the desire to do harm, even to the doctor. And then the doctor has to defend himself.

By the nature of our activity, we pronounce on the diagnoses established by our colleagues from other medical specialties, and situations often arise in which we challenge these diagnoses. The consequences are easy to suspect (conflicts with the patients, with our colleagues from other specialties, who do not know the criteria for medical expertise to the extent that we know the clinical and paraclinical criteria for establishing the medical diagnoses, and even criminal complaints). Our professional training is such that we can always support our resolutions.

But we need the medical expertise not only for malpractice.

People wanted to defend themselves, to protect themselves.

And so humans did 2 things - they invented the insurance and they used the medical expertise, same as the external audit in accountability.

References

1. Soare Ioana, International Pensions - Insurance Medicine, Etna Publishing House, 2010
2. Aurelian Buzăianu, Judicial and extrajudicial technical expertise - Metallurgical products and technologies, 2010, Nomina Lex Publishing House, pg 13, 17
3. www.asim.unibas.ch
4. https://aimj.org/english/
5. www.aaimedicine.org

CHAPTER 2

DOCTORS IN THIS FIELD

IOANA SOARE

The role of "devil's attorney" between the patient and the employer of the doctor is very difficult to sustain. That is why we recommend that the doctor must be self-employed - to be equidistant from these 2 poles of interest. The main role is to advise and examine the patient and to recommend further steps.

There are not only doctors/physicians working in the insurance medicine.

The private sector, faster than the state sector when it comes to cut costs, has parted underwriting (gathering information about the patient) from the rest. They have hired nurses and even personnel with a one-week qualification for asking data per telephone. Only in some Eastern European countries the underwriting is made by doctors, because of the cheap working force. In the USA there are non-physician underwriters.

They have parted also the medical claims to be considered by an economist or a lawyer, called medical claims director/ manager. Only the difficult files are sent to a doctor, and in seldom cases the patient is seen by this doctor. So, in the private sector they evaluate mainly the papers.

In the USA the physicians (MD, DO) practicing Insurance Medicine work within the fields of life, health, disability and long-term care insurance. Medical Directors analyze the medical records of the applicants to determine the insurance risk and to evaluate the life and disability claims. Based upon the current health assessment, a Medical Director predicts the probability of survival many decades into the future.

A number of Medical Directors have training in the Internal Medicine subspecialties such as cardiology, oncology and pulmonary medicine. In addition to a fund of general medical knowledge, Medical Directors receive training on the life expectancy estimation and the risk assessment. Additional training is largely provided on the job. The Medical Directors may be called on to do any of the following:

- Give an opinion, from a medical perspective, if the death of the person was accidental.
- Review the additional information
- Review the claims that occur within the contestable period of a life insurance contract.
- Review the Disability Income (DI) claims or the Waiver of Premium (WP) claims.
- Review the claims with regard to suicide as the cause of death.
- Testify in court or via deposition as a representative of the company or as an expert witness.
- Evaluate the employee disability and the Worker's Compensation claims.
- Consult on the Family Medical Leave Act (FLMA) and the Americans with Disabilities Act (ADA).
- Assess the Long Term Care (LTC), Health Insurance and Critical Illness Claims.

In the US, there are about 500 doctors practicing the Insurance Medicine in the life and disability fields.

In the European Union we have doctors working for the state insurance companies, doing the underwriting and evaluating the medical claims, but they do not always issue a medical decision – in the Czech Republic and Slovakia, the director, an economist most frequently, issues the decision. In the other countries in EU, the insurance doctor gives the medical decision, followed by an administrative decision issued by the economists at the national house of pensions/ state insurance company. In each country there are a few hundred doctors working full time in this field – Romania, 200 medical doctors called insurance medical experts, and in Slovakia, the Czech Republic, about 3-400. There are also much more doctors working part-time.

For the private companies in EU there are not only doctors/ physicians working in this domain.

1. Education

The doctors must study 4 years the insurance medicine in Holland, Belgium and Romania, and together with the legal medicine in Italy, Spain and Portugal. Then they are recognized as medical specialists in the insurance medicine.

Some countries in EU require that the doctor studies and works in another specialty before training 1-3 years in the insurance medicine – Germany, France, Slovakia, the Czech Republic 1 year in France or even 2 weeks in the Great Britain, followed by courses.

Role/Activity

Particularities of the examination – in our area of activity we must examine the patient or the file from a medical point of view, and also from a contractual/legislative point of view.

The medical examination has a few special components, compared to the classical one:

1. we must advise about the insurance rights of the person examined, about his/ her claim

2. we must establish if the diagnostic and the treatment are correct, according to the medical guides respecting the Evidence Based Medicine

3. we must appreciate the evolution and the prognostic, the risk

4. we must check if the patient hides other diagnostics, minimizing them, or if he/ she exaggerates or mimics the present diagnostic

5. we must initiate and even impose the physical and vocational rehabilitation, favorizing the return to work

6. we must evaluate the functional capacity of the patient, related to the daily tasks at home and related to his/ her working place

7. we must issue a medical decision, as in Romania, France, Italy, Belgium, Norway.

CHAPTER 3

ASSOCIATIONS OF MEDICAL DOCTORS WORKING IN INSURANCE MEDICINE

IOANA SOARE

ICLAM - International Committee for Insurance Medicine

The history of **ICLAM** started in 1899, when E. Poëls, Chief Medical Director of Compagnie Belge d´Assurances Générales, organized the first International Conference in Brussels. At the conference, the attendees agreed on the foundation of an international association.

First names:

- Congrès International de Médecins Experts des Compagnies d'Assurances (1899-1906)
- Thanks to doctor Poëls, ICLAM was founded on September 24th 1901 in Amsterdam as the Association Internationale de Médecins Experts des Compagnies d'Assurances (AIMECA). AIMECA was an international association with national committees.
- International Congress of Examining Physicians for Insurance-Companies (1906)
- International Congress for Insurance Medicine (1906).
- After three years of preparation, ICLAM restarted at a special meeting during the 6th International Congress for Accidents and Occupational Diseases, held August 1931 in Geneva. Present at this meeting were the representatives from Germany, the Netherlands, Italy, Sweden, and Switzerland. It was decided that they would form a provisionary Bureau that would prepare the foundation of a new organization, called Permanent International Committee for the study of Life Assurance Medicine, with the representatives from

Belgium, France, Germany, Italy, the Netherlands, Sweden, Switzerland and the United Kingdom.

- Under the direction of F. Kaufman, in Zürich, the acronym **ICLAM** was brought into existence, although the full name was The Permanent International Committee for the study of Life Assurance Medicine. In May 2006 the name was changed to International Committee for Insurance Medicine, but the acronym **ICLAM** still stands as it is well-known and respected.
- Over the years **ICLAM,** which started as an European organization, has expanded to hold conferences on the other continents in keeping with its title.

Now, ICLAM organizes congresses every 2 years in different parts of the world - Berlin, Cape Town, Mumbai, Estoril and others. These scientific manifestations have an important role in the uniformization of the medical practice in insurance medicine.

ICLAM is based in Switzerland.

References

https://www.iclam.org/history/

AMCAP Association des Medecins Conseils en Assurances des Personnes

AMCAP is a scholarly association, grouping the French physicians working in the medical expertise or as advisors for the insurance companies, in the contractual field. The AMCAP, Advising Physicians in Insurance Medicine Association, is involved in the formation and maintenance of specific knowledge of the profession.

They offer the 1year University Diploma in Insurance Medicine. It is awarded by the Faculty of Medicine of Marseilles, under the authority of Professor George Léonetti. It is a third cycle diploma. The courses are delivered by the specialists of the Faculty and by many members of this association. The training lasts one year. It combines the theoretical training courses in medical services companies. It begins in the academic year in October. 60 hours of instruction are delivered by 40 teachers. We have put together this education on THREE DAYS TWO SEMINARS, fairly dense.

The procedures for verification of knowledge:

- Attendance at the seminars is essential
- A continuous assessment using pre and post tests
- An individual oral exam
- An article written by the working groups of 2 to 4 "students".

Training: Every four years, we hope that the oneday seminar will enable to update the knowledge of each and further validation of the diploma.

References

https://www.amcap.fr/

Romanian Societies

1. CMEA, Asociatia profesionala Corpul Medicilor Experti de Asigurari, **Health and Life Insurance Medical Experts Professional Association** was created in 2005 as a Romanian juridical person of private right, non-governmental and non-political, with a non-profit character. **CMEA** was member of EUMASS 2009-2019 and is member of ICLAM since 2007.

The main goal of CMEA is to maintain and perfect a competent, specialized and efficient professional body, in order to protect and promote the professional interests through the following:

- representation of the interests and rights of the health and life insurance medical expert profession in Romania and abroad;
- initiation and support of the profession specific legislative measures, at the central and local state authority level;
- setting up of the Romanian health and life insurance medical experts index and the creation of a central level database containing the health and life insurance medical experts;
- endorsement of the health and life insurance medical experts cohesion based on the professional partnership, solidarity and discipline;
- assertion of the professional body representation at the civil society level and in relation with the state authorities;
- promotion of the expertise and information exchange among its members and with specialized Romanian or foreign organizations;
- organization of the reunions and symposiums of interest for the members, including international participations;
- co-ordination of the studies and researches concerning the health and life insurance medical expert profession;
- publishing of the periodicals and the occasional journals;

- initiation of the training and specialization programs in collaboration with its members;
- endorsement of the reliable solutions for the integration of the health and life insurance medical expert profession;
- endorsement of the sponsoring and management programs to be achieved by members' effort, by complying with the law provisions;
- participation in the international activities (workshops, meetings, congresses, scientific research activities, publication of periodicals and scientific magazines) in the medical field;
- affiliation to the similar national and international bodies;
- promotion of the Association's activities and research results by all mass-media means, publication, printing and distribution of books, magazines, reports, monographs, recommendations, studies and other kind of publications and specialized papers;
- the creation and administration of a documentation, information and distribution centre for the products and services in connection with the Association's goal;
- the creation and awarding of prizes, grants and stimuli for special achievements related to the Association's goal, independently or in collaboration with other organizations;
- the endorsement and support of a modern communication system among the Association's members for their mutual benefit, in order to disseminate the information and knowledge concerning the medical industry.

CMEA has produced an Insurance Physician statute, actually in discussion in the Romanian Parliament.

References

Statute of Health and Life Insurance Medical Experts Professional Association, **CMEA**

2. SREMRCM Romanian Society of Medical Assessment and Work Capacity Rehabilitation

The Romanian Society of Medical Assessment and Work Capacity Rehabilitation (SREMRCM – the Romanian abbreviation) is a scientific and professional organization of the social insurance physicians. With legal personality, this non-profit organization gathers the professionals in the field of the social medicine.

The purpose of the association is to develop the medical assessment of the work capacity by:

- Fostering the scientific research
- Cooperating with the higher education medical institutions and higher education institutions in the connected fields in order to train and specialise the highly-prepared professionals
- Improving the professional and scientific level of its members
- Cooperating with other Romanian or foreign professional, scientific and research institutes in order to prevent the disability
- Establishing a code of professional ethics and ensuring its compliance by the members
- Improving the prestige and representing, supporting and fostering the professional and scientific interests.

In order to reach the purpose for which it was established, the Association "Romanian Society of Medical Assessment and Work Capacity Rehabilitation" may have the following activities:

- Organising the National Conference of the social insurance physicians in Romania, the congresses, deliberations and symposia and participating by delegation in any medical scientific events in Romania or abroad
- Organising the scientific research sessions
- Publishing papers in the journals of the field
- Organising, together with the sectors of the field, courses or research studies
- Obtaining angel investments or subsidies
- Granting prizes or honours for the young doctors' exceptional professional and scientific activity
- Editing and disseminating the Romanian Journal of Medical Assessment and Work Capacity Rehabilitation, which is distributed to the specialist doctors at the Congress or meetings
- Cooperating with the Ministry of Health in the activity of health protection (the medical aid and the scientific research)
- Disseminating the main conclusions of various scientific events as well as certain suggestions for the regulations that do not exist in the active legislation to the Ministry of Labour, Ministry of Health, the Academy of Medical Sciences and other similar institutions that will materialise them in the future

- Affiliating with the international specialised organizations and cooperating with the similar foreign societies.

SREMRCM is a EUMASS member since 2009.

References

https://sremrcm.ro/ro/

UEMASS / EUMASS Union Européene de Médecine d'Assurance et de Sécurité Sociale / European Union of Medicine in Assurance and Social Security

FOUNDATION - 1972. Orleans, France – Meeting of French Medical Advisers. The French medical director, Claude Persignan and a Belgian observer, René Rénard, discussed the idea of an organization of the Medical Advisers, of the then existing Common Market countries, to promote the scientific and social exchanges between the member states.

1973. The Founding Convention, München, Germany. The signatories were representatives of Belgium, France, Germany, Italy, Luxembourg and the Netherlands. The first Congress was held in 1974, in Brussels, Belgium.

ENLARGEMENT

1992: UK became a full member in 1992. Italy was represented again in 1996, and there has been Italian involvement in all subsequent projects.

1996: Membership of the representative organizations of Ireland, Sweden, and Norway, the first non-EU country to join.

1999: Representatives of the Czech Republic and Hungary joined the Council.

OBJECTIVES - EUMASS-UEMASS coordinates the exchange of information between the countries in relation to the social insurance medicine. The association organizes congresses every 2 years.

EUMASS-UEMASS represents social insurance doctors (some working also in private insurance companies) at the European level, not in any political or economic sense, but as a body that is able to generate ideas, initiate studies, compare results of work experiences, consider suggestions, and disseminate the information through publications.

EUMASS-UEMASS helps to maintain and improve the standards in the social insurance medicine.

The international nature of the big commercial enterprises and the migration of the employees within the European Union, linked to the increased involvement of the private sector in the social insurance medicine in some countries, already generates work on the international comparisons on medical services.

The disability assessment presents many of the same challenges in social insurance and private insurance medical work. EUMASS encourages the links between the doctors working for the social insurance and the private insurance organizations.

Special membership is available to the occupational physicians, general practitioners, academics, and any others who have an involvement in the healthcare or disability assessment. This membership is on an individual basis, on application to the Council.

The Working Groups - EUMASS-UEMASS has two spheres of interest - the DISABILITY MEDICAL ASSESSMENT and HEALTHCARE COST CONTROL. In countries where healthcare cost-control falls outside the remit of the social insurance, representatives try to encourage the participation of the relevant organizations, so that the information can still be shared.

UEMASS/EUMASS was based in Belgium, now it is based in Switzerland.

References

www.eumass.org

AAIM

The American Academy of Insurance Medicine (AAIM) was founded in 1889, as 34 physicians from 27 insurance companies formed the Association of Life Insurance Medical Directors of America (ALIMDA) in New York.

ALIMDA addressed all professional medical interests relating to the risk selection, including the studies, education, professional and public relations. In 1991 the name was changed to the American Academy of Insurance Medicine (AAIM).

In the 19th century the physicians conducted medical examinations to ensure that life insurance was offered only to those who seemed to be healthy. The existence of a professional organization promoted the development of consistency and fairness in the risk selection process. ALIMDA also encouraged the application of the medico-actuarial methodology to make the underwriting more scientific. By the end of the century, the early life insurance research had demonstrated the mortality implications of the results of routine urinalysis for protein and sugar. This proved to be a valuable contribution to both insurance and clinical medicine.

Throughout the past century the medico-actuarial studies were conducted by the medical directors and actuaries within companies and with multi-company data in conjunction with actuarial associations. Notable contributions have included the Build and Blood Pressure Study published intermittently from 1925 through 1979. In the 1950s these studies were the first to show conclusively that the elevated blood pressure determines an increased mortality.

Insurance for the individuals with medical impairments was made possible by a numerical rating system devised in 1919. This substandard risk rating system has since made the life insurance widely available to many people with health problems.

From the beginning, the educational needs of the insurance medical directors have been addressed at the annual meetings. Guest experts from the academic medicine and from the insurance industry discussed the advances in medicine and their application to the risk assessment process. In the 1960s ALIMDA also created the Board of Insurance Medicine (BIM) that has established the criteria for diplomat recognition. The BIM developed an intensive and comprehensive triennial course in insurance medicine that continues today as a key educational source.

The 1960s saw the birth of the Journal of Insurance Medicine. This respected journal is published quarterly and focuses on the mortality and morbidity analysis of the medical and insurance research.

Our physician members typically serve as medical directors to the insurance companies. Members may serve these companies as advisors for underwriting and consultants for the claims and disability management. Other roles include the medical and actuarial research, the underwriting guideline development, the employee health education and care, and as the professional liaison to the medical community, legislative bodies and regulatory agencies.

AAIM maintains the commitment to education and research started by ALIMDA over a century ago. It has created associate and affiliate memberships for those involved with the insurance medicine who are not employed as medical directors of the insurance companies. AAIM continues to address the many professional and public relations interests of the insurance medical community, including the ongoing representation in the American Medical Association.

References

https://aaimedicine.org/about-aaim/history-of-aaim.asp, visited 14.12.2024

PART 4

ASSESSMENT/ PATIENT EVALUATION

CHAPTER 1

INSURANCE UNDERWRITING

IOANA SOARE

The term "underwrite" originates in the 17th century when the marine vessels would be underwritten for the insurance risk for the overseas voyages. The employee of the insurance company would sub-scribe (literally to write underneath or under-write) the policy by signing their name at the bottom of the document and acknowledging the consent that the policy is in force [1].

Underwriting is the process of evaluating the patient's right to the type of insurance and his risks. It also applies in the banking field, when the individual applies for a loan [1]. Literally it means that somebody (an expert) has evaluated the claim and the risk and has signed the papers.

The insurance companies have a policy for granting the loans/insurance policies. Depending on this approach, some patients may be accepted and some not, and if the risk is high, the patient will pay extra for the insurance. In general, the insured must be distributed, from a statistical point of view, on the Gaussian curve. Not all young and healthy, not all very old or very sick. Thus, the profitability of the company is balanced [1].

Underwriting is a process that involves:

- Acceptance of the risk
- Risk evaluation
- Risk acceptance
- Risk pricing
- Application of the policy conditions
- Exposure management [1].

With the insurance underwriting, the focus is on the potential policyholder—the person seeking the health or life insurance. In the past, the medical underwriting for health insurance was used to determine how much to charge an applicant based on their health and even whether to offer coverage at all, often based on the applicant's pre-existing conditions. Beginning in 2014, under the Affordable Care Act, the insurers were no longer allowed to deny coverage or impose limitations based on the pre-existing conditions [2].

Life insurance underwriting seeks to assess the risk of insuring a potential policyholder based on their age, health, lifestyle, occupation, family medical history, hobbies, and other factors determined by the underwriter. Life insurance underwriting can result in the approval—along with a range of coverage amounts, prices, exclusions, and conditions—or outright rejection [1].

Life insurance policies are more complicated because they also account for the insured's medical history. Underwriting life insurance can take a month or longer, although most decisions are issued in a few days [3].

For life insurance, they might also look at their medical history, including the risk factors such as smoking or drinking [4].

A big part of the underwriter's job is to weigh the known risk factors and investigate an applicant's truthfulness to determine the minimum price for providing coverage.

References

1. http://www.investinganswers.com/financial-dictionary/insurance/underwriting-1545 visited 23.05.2016
2. Banton Caroline, Underwriting: Definition and How the Various Types Work, https://www.investopedia.com/terms/u/underwriting.asp#toc-how-underwriting-works, updated December 19, 2023, visited 28.06.2024
3. Independent Insurance Agents & Brokers of America. "Underwriting Period by State, https://www.independentagent.com/vu/SiteAssets/Reference%20Lists/Underwriting-Period-by-State.pdf
4. Guardian Life. "Life Insurance Underwriting: What To Expect." https://www.guardianlife.com/life-insurance/underwriting

CHAPTER 2

PATIENT ASSESSMENT

IOANA SOARE

Self-Evaluation

In UK, Department of Work and Pensions approved questionnaires for self-evaluation. In difficult cases, the patient is examined by medical personnel.

There are some older attempts to self-evaluation, as the Australian SF36 Questionnaire, more elaborate, and the European EuroQol- 5 Dimension (EQ-5D), mostly used for evaluating the generic quality of life and not in Life insurance.

Other self-administered questionnaires are used in diagnostic.

Physician evaluation

Why we do not examine only the papers?

Why should the patient be examined?

1. Because he can declare diseases he does not have.
2. Because he can hide diseases he has.
3. Because he may have diseases he dosn't know he has [1].

It will be done from a clinical, paraclinical, psychological and social point of view [2,3].

Patient expertise involves three stages:

a) a direct, complete clinical consultation of the patient or/and consultation of the medical documentation, the result of this stage being the confirmation or the denial of the diagnoses established by our colleagues in any other medical specialty. Obviously, at this stage we have direct contact with the patients, many of whom have infectious-contagious diseases or mental illnesses, which represent a great professional risk for us (tuberculosis, AIDS, schizophrenia or other delusional disorders, etc.).

b) the evaluation of a functional diagnosis, from which the establishment of disability or work capacity can then be derived (respectively adaptive incapacity and the degree of disability), from the International Classification of Functionality and Disability, ICF, point of view [2]. This stage ends with the issuance of a decision on work capacity, a disability certificate or other forms, on the basis of which people usually receive money (pension, allowance, benefit, compensatory payment). The papers can be used to obtain other insurance benefits - as in the case of disability, road accidents, work accidents or occupational diseases.

c) the establishment of a recovery plan, through which the patient is guided on the measures to be taken to improve or even cure his ailments, the purpose of this stage being the recovery of the work capacity, re-employment or social reintegration [1].

The evaluation involves a rigorous and detailed clinical examination, which begins the moment the patient enters the office door:

- How he/she/it walks (hesitantly, slowly, leaning), how he sits on the chair (slowly, leaning on the table)
- How he/she/it answers questions
- How he/she/it undresses
- The shape of the head, body and limbs
- The colour of the face, lips, ears, eyes conjunctiva

Examination of the head

Place both palms on the top of the patient's head and gently palpate the skull with all fingers, then palpate the face, where the cranial nerves exit subcutaneously - above and below the eyebrows, paranasal, on the sinuses, pre - and behind the ears, on the mandible. Palpate the eyes very gently, bilaterally (to detect pressure differences). The pupillary reflex must be taken. The patient is asked to look at the doctor's finger, up-down, left-right.

We will ask the patient to open the mouth, stick out the tongue. We will evaluate the missing teeth, the present dental works - it tells us the patient's anxiety towards the dentist and the economic level.

We palpate the temporomandibular joints, also in motion, to detect painful points on the joint line, anatomical changes, swings or subluxations that may indicate a higher dental work on one side.

We bilaterally palpate the Arnold points at the occipital level, then the mastoid, the parotid glands, the chains of pre and retro sternocleidomastoid nodes, the thyroid and the supraclavicular fossa [1].

Examination of the upper limbs

We simultaneously palpate the muscles of the shoulders, arms and forearms bilaterally. Left and right differences may appear after fractures. The feeling of stretched or weak muscle are encountered in the enzyme deficiencies with genetic determinism.

We examine the movements in each joint, symmetrically, simultaneously.

We examine the force of prehension - with our right hand we test the right hand - the thumb-index clamp, then thumb-finger 3, etc., then the left hand. Decreased strength in certain segments may indicate a severe neurological deficit.

We palpate the pulse in both hands at the level of the radial artery - weak/strong, regular, irregular.

We count the heartbeats for 30 seconds. We count the extrasystoles, if any - they are significant above 6/min. The blood pressure is taken in both arms - only the higher one is taken into account [1].

Chest examination

The axillary nodes are then palpated, with the patient's hands resting on the hips, to highlight the tip of the axilla. The doctor then washes his hands. After asking for consent, also in men, women, other, palpate the mammary glands, in quarters, from the center to the periphery and then from top down and from the outside to the inside.

The respiratory movements and costal excursions are examined (we make the patient breathe deeply while holding the hands on the intercostal spaces).

The lungs are auscultated behind, laterally, symmetrically, then on the front of the chest.

The heart is auscultated first on the anterior left axillary line VI-VII space, then submammar, then IV space left latero-sternal, then right; latero-sternal space II-III left, then left latero-cervical and then right, for carotid murmurs.

Examination of the abdomen

Visually examine the abdomen for scars, hernias, or eventrations. Ask the patient to cough. Palpate the abdomen from the lower left to the lower right, first superficially, then deeply.

Examination of the lumbar and sacral region

Palpate the lumbar muscles, from bottom to top, in parallel, simultaneously. The lateral hernial triangle must be checked.

The lumbar spinous apophyses are percussed. Slow percussion is made with the side of the palm on the renal areas. We press gently on the last ribs. The sacral holes and the Valleix points on the gluteal muscles are palpated.

Examination of the lower limbs

We bilaterally palpate the muscles of the hips, thighs and calves.

We examine the movements in each joint, symmetrically, simultaneously. The Lasegue maneuver is performed.

We palpate the knees, ankles and fingers.

We check the pulse at the level of the pediotic artery bilaterally.

A short neurological examination must be performed - walking (toe-toe, heel-toe), Romberg test, reflexes, skin sensitivity.

Then questions are asked to the patient, WITHOUT SUGGESTING THE ANSWER.

When do you get dizzy? (when getting up from the armchair or bed, when driving...)

How are your feet in bed at night? (Cold or warm)

Where do you keep your feet at night - under the covers or out? (hyperthyroidism, hyper...)

When does your chest hurt? Day/night, when do you walk or when do you stay?

Repeat small questions about personal data.

Ask questions about past events.

These questions guide us regarding the psychological status (recent memory, attention, decay coefficient).

In mentally ill patients, avoid the irritant focus - it's the job of the psychiatrist. But if it's stable, chronic, you can ask if he/she/it has ever heard voices and if they were benevolent or not. He can also be asked how he gets along with his relatives and neighbors.

Show the patient some documents and ask how old they are. This is how we test vision. You can ask him also to read your handwriting.

Evaluation exception

The medical and psychological examination of personnel with attributions in transport safety are approved by law in many countries (the Ministry of Transport and Ministry of Health - in Romania).

Conclusion

One way of dealing with the susceptibility to bias of assessment interviews is to use protocols for interviewing the claimants. In the Dutch practice several such protocols have been developed. These protocols correspond with concepts in the ICF and the biopsychosocial approach. There is a professional consensus among experienced Dutch SIPs about the principle of assessment on arguments, the principle of conducting a semi-structured interview and the most crucial interview topics, which cover all fields of ICF [4].

References

1. Soare Ioana, Medical Expertise, Insurance Medicine, Handbook for the General Medicine Faculty, 2017, Etna Publishing House, pg 27-68
2. http://apps.who.int/iris/bitstream/10665/42407/5/9241545429_rum.pdf, published by WHO in 2001
3. Council of Europe: Assessing disability in Europe. Strasbourg 2002.

4. de Boer WE, Wind H, van Dijk FJ, Willems HH. Interviews for the assessment of long-term incapacity for work: a study on adherence to protocols and principles. BMC Public Health. 2009 Jun 2;9: 169. doi: 10.1186/1471-2458-9-169. PMID: 19490614; PMCID: PMC2698854.

CHAPTER 3

ASSESSING PATIENTS WITH RARE DISEASES

IOANA SOARE

Introduction

The assessment of any patient is based on the International Classification of Functioning, Disability and Health, ICF. Thus we evaluate people with extremely different diseases, based on the percentage of the functional deficit [1].

There are over 6000 diseases considered rare, 72% having genetic origins [2].

At the EU level, there is EURORDIS, the European network dedicated exclusively to the rare diseases. Recently the UN established an International Committee for Rare Diseases, precisely to emphasize their importance and the situations, the legal relationships and the medical problems these patients generate [2].

In the European Union, even if there are few patients of each disease in each country, in total we estimate 30 million people affected by rare diseases, diseases that are difficult to diagnose and treat [2].

In each country there is specific legislation. Also, at the European level, there are two Directives, 24/2011, respectively 89/1988 and the Council Recommendation (2009/c 151/02).

Globally, the management of each rare disease is carried out by the networks of Centers of Expertise in the Field of Rare Diseases.

A European Register of rare diseases, Rare Disease Platform, has also recently been implemented.

Because these patients have lost between 3 and 7 years until they were diagnosed, the centers of excellence were established to facilitate their guidance and treatment, such as the Center of Excellence in Hematological Diseases at the Bucharest University Emergency Hospital.

The civil society, through the associations and foundations, has the merit of supporting these people with special needs. The lobbying carried out and the pressure exerted have materialized in a wider awareness and support given to the sick [3,4].

To better describe the rare disorders of genetic origin, Orphanet provides information on each gene linked to a rare disorder. [5]. This information includes international genetic nomenclature, gene typology (gene with protein product, locus, non-coding RNA), chromosomal location, and cross-mapping with the international genetic databases.

A rare disease requires a circuit of medical investigations, evaluation criteria in terms of disability, social inclusion, and rights of the patient, a great social responsibility. Because the scarce data, Directive 24/2011 regulates and encourages cross-border medicine and requires the implementation of the Community acquis, to ensure a clear legal framework.

The patient must be supported and his special needs met, within the limits of the acceptance of the society in which we live.

Assessment

The medical exam must assess the symptoms, the extent and evolution of the disease and the effects of the treatment, but also to determine the functional deficit and the special needs of the patient.

A patient's health status is examined according to the ICF from the physical (body functions, structures), mental (activities and participation) and social (environmental, contextual factors – e.g. poverty, rural areas) points of view. Each factor can act as a facilitator or as an obstacle in the patient's social integration [6].

Apart from the impairment of the body's functions (for example reduced vision, deafness, heart failure) and the modification of structures (for example the lack of a kidney, a limb due to amputation), I detail factors less evaluated by the specialist physician.

Activities and participation:

- Basic learning and applying it
    - Sensory experiences
- General tasks and requests
- Communication
- Mobility
- Self-care
- Self-management
- Interpersonal interactions and relationships
- Major areas of life
- Community, civic and social life

The functional impairment is equivalent to disability, from the point of view of the researchers that developed ICF.

From the point of view of the insurance physician a human is considered normal, if the functional deficiency is below 30% (just as we appreciate the normal on Nomograms in spirometry, for example) [6].

Conclusions

"You can have only one patient with a certain disease in a country. He has the right by the Constitution (in Romania) to health. We can't say: your treatment is too expensive, we won't pay for it." Dorica Dan, President of the Romanian Association of Rare Cancers [3].

6000 rare diseases, one common denominator – the functional impairment and one support – EURORDIS.

References

1. Soare Ioana, Medical expertise – Insurance medicine, 2017, Etna Publishing House, Bucharest
2. https://www.eurordis.org/IMG/pdf/RO-Eurordis-Presentation-Colour.pdf
3. https://www.arcrareromania.ro/
4. https://www.bolirareromania.ro/sites/default/files/politici/PNBR%202014-2020.pdf
5. https://www.orpha.net/consor/cgi-bin/Disease_Genes.php?lng=EN

6. CIF, http://anpd.gov.ro/web/wp-content/uploads/2016/06/Classificationa-internationala-a-functionarii-dizabilitatii-si-sanatatii-CIF-CT-versiunea-pentru-copii- and-youth-2012.

CHAPTER 4

THE EUMASS CORE SET FOR DISABILITY ASSESSMENT

IOANA SOARE

In 2004, the EUMASS council established a working group on ICF to develop a **core set for functional evaluation in disability**. This core set could offer a practical starting base for uniformization of disability evaluation in EU. The working group selected 20 categories: five for body functions and 15 for activities and participation.

In 2015 this core set was published in "Handbook of Vocational Rehabilitation and Disability Evaluation", named as the **EUMASS core set for disability evaluation**. It has been used as a basis for the development of procedures in Sweden, France, the Netherlands and Iceland.

EUMASS Core set for disability evaluation in social security

Code	Title
b164	Higher-level cognitive functions
b280	Sensation of pain
b455	Exercise tolerance functions
b710	Mobility of joint functions
b730	Muscle power functions
d110	Watching
d115	Listening
d155	Acquiring skills
d177	Making decisions
d220	Undertaking multiple tasks
d240	Handling stress and other psychological demands

d399	Communication, unspecified
d410	Changing basic body position
d415	Maintaining a body position
d430	Lifting and carrying objects
d440	Fine hand use
d445	Hand and arm use
d450	Walking
d470	Using transportation
d720	Complex interpersonal interactions

[1]

Reference

1. https://www.eumass.eu/wp-content/uploads/2016/10/Brage.pdf

CHAPTER 5

IMPORTANCE OF THE SOCIAL DETERMINANTS OF HEALTH IN ASSESSMENT (SDOH)

IOANA SOARE

Introduction

The World Health Organization (WHO) imposed, since 1980, a new bio-psycho-social model for the patient evaluation in based on ICF. This was connected to the new definition of health, also implemented by WHO, as "a state of complete physical, mental and social well-being and not merely the absence of disease and infirmity" [1,2].

Prof. Rachel Rowe, School of Population Health, Australia, published in Big Data & Society, July–December: 1–12, SAGE, an article regarding SDOH. She stated: In recent years, the claim that around 80 percent of contemporary health issues are attributable to social factors has become a mantra at digital health technology conferences [3].

The Public Health Agency of Canada has identified 12 determinants of health [4]:

- Income and social status
- Social support networks
- Education and literacy
- Employment / working conditions
- Social environments
- Physical environments
- Personal health practices and coping skills
- Healthy development of the child
- Biology and genetic endowment
- Health services
- Sex

υ Culture.

An important role in the evaluation of the claim should be imposed by the social factors. The medical model of disability is first assessed, but the social model may surge out.

The evaluation of the literature, focusing on medical-social factors, so far only considered contextual to the health, showed great impact of the education level, marital status, behavioral factors (smoking) on the quality of life and professional insertion of the patients [5].

Social factors may be more important in determining the unemployment and the disability retirement than the medical factors [5].

Conclusions

All these social factors have derived from statistical observations.

In private insurance companies, most of these factors were considered for a long time ago.

The first international important report was the Commission on Social Determinants of Health FINAL REPORT – WHO 2008. The Healthy People 2020 Approach to Social Determinants of Health is another report developed by WHO.

Considering all these, we can say that the modern tendencies are towards the medico-social guidelines in the insurance medicine.

References

1. Leonardi M, Lee H, Kostanjsek N, et al. 20 Years of ICF-International Classification of Functioning, Disability and Health: Uses and Applications around the World. Int J Environ Res Public Health. **2022**;19(18):11321. doi: 10.3390/ijerph191811321
2. Švestková O, Sládková P, Kotková K. Application of International Classification of Functioning, Disability and Health (ICF), Functional Health and Disability. Cent Eur J Public Health. **2016**;24(1):83-5. doi: 10.21101/cejph.a4140
3. Rowe R. Social determinants of health in the Big Data mode of population health risk calculation. Big Data & Society, **2021**;8(2). doi: 10.1177/20539517211062881

4. Lucyk K. Intersectoral action on the social determinants of health and health equity in Canada: December 2019 federal government mandate letter review. Health Promot Chronic Dis Prev Can. 2020 Oct; 40(10):314-323. doi: 10.24095/hpcdp.40.10.03
5. Frank J, Abel T, Campostrini S, Cook S, Lin VK, McQueen DV. The Social Determinants of Health: Time to Re-Think? Int J Environ Res Public Health. 2020 Aug 12;17(16):5856. doi: 10.3390/ijerph17165856.

CHAPTER 6

DISABILITY ASSESSMENT IN GREAT BRITAIN (UK)

VALENTIN EUGEN CIOCSAN

There is no sickness pension in the UK. There is only early retirement, regardless of cause. In the case of health problems that cause disabilities, the state grants a distinct financial aid, unrelated to the person's status: active or retired.

Here, the family doctor (general practitioner, GP) is not obliged to formulate a diagnosis. They send the patient to a specialist (the most appropriate), mentioning only the symptoms and signs, possibly the suspicion. That, of course, apart from common diseases that are easy to identify after some simple investigations. Medical practice is analyzed only by the professional body, directly the General Council of Doctors (GMC), without any intrusion from the Department of Health. Since 1948, the State healthcare has been completely free - this does not mean that it is somehow of lower quality, only that the waiting time is longer compared to private services (but not in the case of emergencies). Until recently, the way to analyze the ability to work, and the ability to manage independently in daily activities, were approached differently.

Today they have been joined as personal independence payment (personal independence allowance) a financial aid for those with disabling health problems who require permanent help or support from another person(s).

The person concerned (or a relative, family member or friend) must complete a form quite detailed, about the disease/diseases that are responsible for their disability and the underlying effects.

From the point of view of the assessor (who previously went through the form), the diagnosis does not constitute everything, apart from obviously disabling conditions (for example in the case of terminal conditions, serious diseases with a poor prognosis, neurological diseases known to cause irreversible damage, those with few sequelae likely to be corrected with prostheses, physiotherapy or other usual means, etc.). The history of the type of activity performed before is less important. The possibility of the patient to perform any activity that would provide him with an income is considered (for example, retraining in another type of job)

When visiting the person, is the main principle, the assessment gathers more detailed information regarding the duration of the illness, the level of care required, possible hospitalizations, instances where an ambulance intervention was necessary, the type of medication followed - and, more importantly, to what extent helps the medication - by the evolution of the condition/conditions causing the reported effects.

A daily life history follows. That's not to say you're curious about what the person is doing. Simple questions: do you sleep well? Do you need help getting out of bed? can you eat alone Why not? Can you handle yourself in the bathroom? How about going up and down stairs (we're in the UK!)? Can you make your own breakfast, lunch, dinner, etc.? Why can't you? And there would be more to describe (continence problems, for example). Next comes the most exhaustive description of mobility (what seem to be the reasons causing these difficulties, are they permanent or how often do they occur?) and the rest of the activities requiring physical effort.

Regarding mental disorders, the assessor mostly follows behaviour, the ability to communicate, relate, the ability to adapt in crowded places or not, the ability to perform simple mental operations. In the case of mental illnesses known to have serious, critical effects, the frequency of crises, their duration, the level of medical assistance, possible hospitalizations, the tendency to harm themselves, suicide attempts, serious antisocial acts, the spatial-temporal orientation are important. We consider the need for supervision and/or assistance with daily activities.

Nota bene: in the case of deafness or mutism, the ability to communicate in BSL (British Sign Language). For the blind, apart from the white ball cane, there are permanent adaptations (auditory signals) in all public places. And on the issue of mobility, there are ramps for those in and out of wheelchairs everywhere. All these adaptations and supports are considered at the assessment, of course, to what extent the persons concerned can use them without help/supervision from someone else.

When it seems necessary, a targeted examination is also done (here you rarely touch the patient without his consent). In the case of mental illnesses, some basic mental tests are performed.

In the description recorded afterwards, you must describe how the person presented during the assessment: difficulties with mobility, general appearance, need for help from a relative, obvious difficulties with respiratory function, safety and strength to perform simple activities during the interview. It assesses the ability to communicate (without considering the need for an interpreter), the expression, attention and apparent cognitive level, signs of obvious stress – essentially how the physical and mental effects of the reported condition(s) appear.

The assessor - here I must specify that he does not necessarily have to be a doctor (here the term medic is used usually for paramedics), he can also be a specially trained assistant. The distribution of cases is made according to the nature and complexity of the condition/conditions reported to be the cause of the reported disability/disabilities.

The assessor must produce an as credible, detailed and convincing a description of the level of disability reported. This must be perfectly sustainable from a medical point of view, that what is reported is credible and has logical support from the point of view of medical practice. The arguments must be entirely consistent.

The report, in 100% proportion, must not contain specialized medical terms. Everything is written in plain English. Why? Because the final decision makers are government officials, basically employees of the DWP (Department for Work and Pensions). The great difficulty of assessors is to draw up a perfectly sustainable image before the professional body, but also convincing for an official without medical training.

Such an assessment generally takes about 30-45 minutes.

Home visits are also made upon reasonably requests. And they follow the same principles.

CHAPTER 7

DISABILITY IN THE USA

IOANA SOARE

Disability is the presence of a condition that makes it more difficult for someone to participate in activities and the world around them. People with disabilities in the U.S. have higher rates of many chronic health conditions and are more likely to have a fall [1]. Chronic diseases and injuries from falls are one of the leading causes of death and disabilities in the USA [2].

Disability has three dimensions:

1. Impairment in a person's mental or physical structure or function
2. Activity limitations that impact life
3. Participation restrictions in daily tasks

In the United States, 61 million adults experience a disability [3].

Social Security manages two disability benefits programs: Social Security Disability, or SSD (a part of Social Security's Old Age, Survivors, and Disability Insurance--OASDI), and Supplemental Security Income, or SSI (which is not paid out of Social Security taxes or the Social Security trust fund).

Social Security Disability Insurance (SSDI). SSDI is a program designed for people who have worked and paid taxes into the Social Security system for years prior to becoming disabled. If an individual is judged disabled, the individual will receive SSDI benefits regardless of the individual's assets or family income [4].

Supplemental Security Income (SSI). SSI, unlike SSDI, is a "needs-based" program. SSI is designed to pay benefits to disabled people who need help with basic living costs, even if they haven't worked or paid taxes into the Social Security system [4,5].

Both programs use the same definition of disability: the inability to work at a full-time job for at least a year due to a serious medical condition. The key to getting approved for disability benefits is to have the proper documentation from the doctor about physical and mental limitations and supporting clinical or laboratory test results. Social Security will look at how much you're working, whether your medical condition matches one of its disability listings, and whether you have the remaining "functional capacity" to do any type of job, even a physically or mentally simple job.

References

1. Centers for Disease Control and Prevention. Disability and Health Related Conditions, https://www.cdc.gov/ncbddd/disabilityandhealth/relatedconditions.html
2. Centers for Disease Control and Prevention. National Center for Health Statistics. FastStats: Leading Causes of Death, https://www.cdc.gov/nchs/fastats/leading-causes-of-death.htm
3. Centers for Disease Control and Prevention. Prevalence of Disabilities and Health Care Access by Disability Status and Type Among Adults—United States, 2016. Morbility and Mortality Weekly Report, https://www.cdc.gov/mmwr/volumes/67/wr/mm6732a3.htm
4. https://www.disabilitysecrets.com/topics/social-security-disability-basics.htm
5. Social Security Administration. Understanding Supplemental Security Income (SSI) Eligibility Requirements. 2022, https://www.ssa.gov/ssi/text-eligibility-ussi.htm#disabled-adult

CHAPTER 8

RESPIRATORY POLYGRAPHY: A KEY ELEMENT IN THE DIAGNOSIS OF BREATHING DISORDERS DURING SLEEP

ȘTEFAN SĂNDULACHE, CONSTANTIN GHIMUȘ AND PARASCHIVA POSTOLACHE

Breathing disorders during the sleep bring together a group of ventilatory disorders, that are becoming more and more common in the medical practice, as a result of the increased level of information and awareness of this pathology, both among professionals and patients.

Breathing disorders during sleep have the potential to generate or exacerbate severe chronic conditions, especially cardiovascular, metabolic and cerebrovascular, and have profoundly unfavourable implications both on the duration and quality of the person's life, as well as on the general demand for medical services, in continuous growth [1,2].

In Romania, the morbidity due to the chronic diseases and, in particular, that due to breathing disorders during sleep remain partially known, due to reasons related to the current information system in the field of health. Moreover, the respiratory pathology, generally associated with other chronic comorbidities, is addressed both in the primary care and in the specialty services, by the physicians from a wide range of medical specialties - the multidisciplinary approach [3]. In this context, there is a heterogeneity of medical practice in both the diagnosis and the clinical management of these diseases.

Somnology is the medical science that deals with the diagnosis and treatment of conditions occurring during sleep.

The American Academy of Sleep Medicine, using the International Classification of Sleep Disorders (3rd edition), divides them into six categories: insomnia, sleep-disordered breathing (figure 1), central hypersomnolence disorders, circadian rhythm sleep-wake disorders, parasomnias, and sleep-related movements [4].

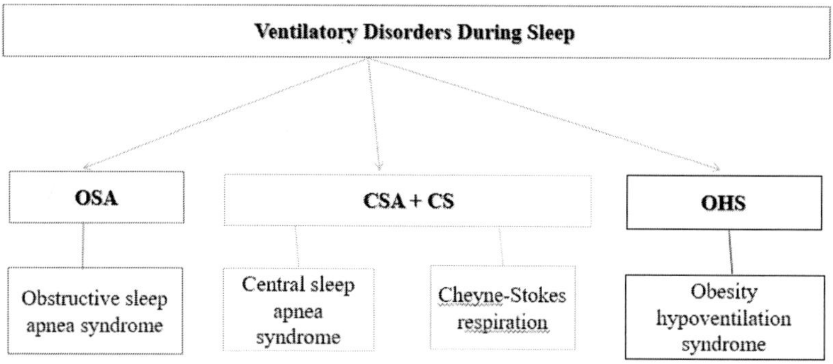

Figure 1. Ventilatory disorders during sleep according to the American Academy of Sleep Medicine [4]

During sleep, the patency of the upper airways is maintained by the balance between their dilator muscles and the negative intraluminal pressure during inspiration. Apnoea is caused by different degrees of narrowing of the upper respiratory tract, determined either by an anatomical defect or by a muscle hypotonia, leading to a narrowing of the upper airways, an increase in their resistance to the air flow and their total (apnoea) or partial (hypopnea) obstruction [5].

Obstructive sleep apnoea syndrome is manifested by recurrent episodes of complete (apnoea) or partial (hypopnea) respiratory collapse during sleep, lasting more than 10 seconds, more than 5/hour of sleep, accompanied by micro-awakenings, >3% decrease in oxygen (hypoxemia) compared to the initial and significant oscillations of the intrathoracic pressure, all of which affect the activity of the sympathetic nervous system, blood pressure and heart rate. The algorithm of the patient with obstructive sleep apnoea syndrome is presented in figure 2 [2].

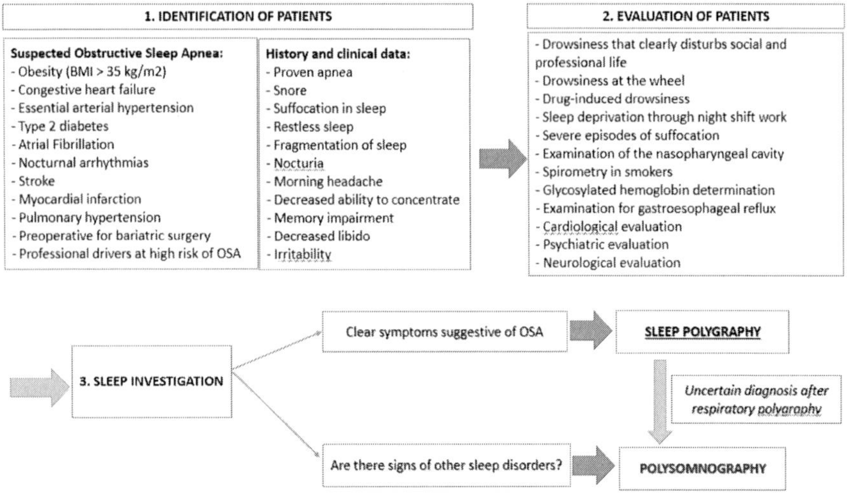

Figure 2. Algorithm of the patient with Obstructive Sleep Apnoea Syndrome

Although the diagnostic gold-standard in sleep apnoea is polysomnography, the small number of laboratories and the high cost of the investigation determined the use of a simpler, cheaper and less laborious method for the diagnosis of obstructive sleep apnoea syndrome. The respiratory polygraph represents the continuous recording, during one night, of the following parameters:

- naso-oral air flow;
- snoring;
- heart rate;
- thoraco-abdominal respiratory effort;
- arterial oxygen saturation;
- body position.

For the detection of periods of apnoea and hypopnea, the polygraph method is as effective as polysomnography, but the lack of an electroencephalogram (EEG) does not allow the correlation of breathing disorders with sleep stages [6].

Polygraph electronic devices (figure 3) define respiratory events (apnoea and hypopnea) based on three basic signals: respiratory flow (assessed by a nasal pressure cannula), inspiratory effort (measured by chest straps) and pulse oximetry [7].

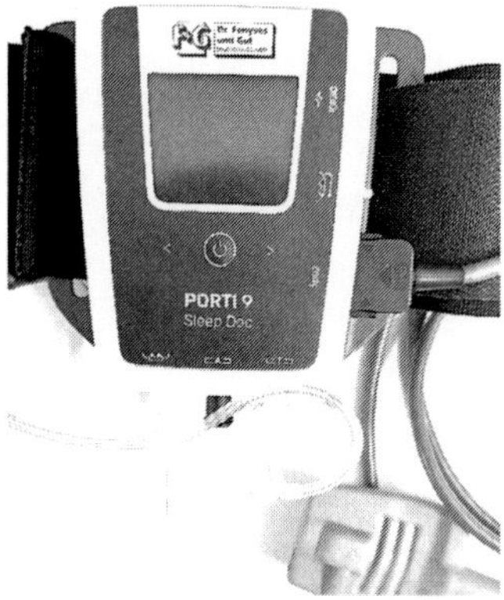

Figure 3. Electronic device for respiratory polygraph recording [Photo Source: Personal Archive]

Rules for correcting sleep tracks regarding polygraph assessment [8]

A) Hypopnea

A respiratory event will be classified as hypopnea if it meets all of the following criteria:

- decrease in peak respiratory flow signal ≥ 30% compared to baseline breathing
- the duration of the fall must be ≥ 10 seconds.
- the presence of oxygen desaturation ≥ 4% (more specific) in relation to the pre-event saturation (figure 4).

If a respiratory event meets the criteria for hypopnea but, in addition, part of it also meets the criteria for apnoea, the entire event should be classified as apnoea.

The presence of hypopnea is particularly important, and sometimes it becomes difficult to identify the beginning and end of the event. Hypopnea begins at the bottom of the first breath with ≥ 30% decrease from the baseline breath and ends at the lowest part of the first breath that equals or exceeds the baseline breath.

Desaturation must be maintained for at least two consecutive seconds.

If the study were conducted with supplemental oxygen, the desaturations could be "attenuated". This information must be mentioned in the report.

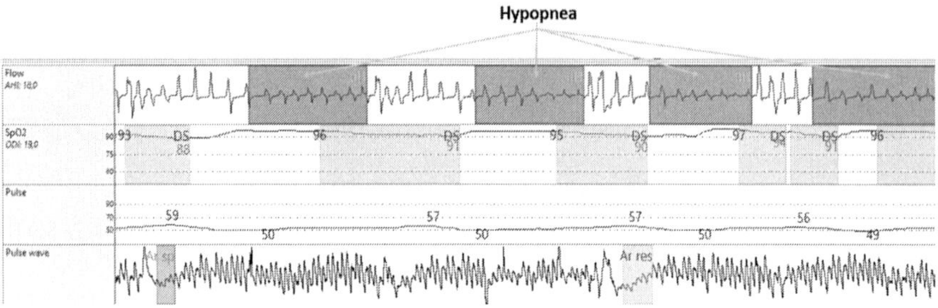

Figure 4. Hypopnea [Photo Source: Personal Archive]

B) Apnoea

A respiratory event is classified as apnoea when the following two criteria are met:

- decrease in the peak respiratory flow signal ≥ 90% compared to the baseline flow, i.e. it is the absence or near absence of breathing.
- the duration of the signal drop must be ≥ 10 seconds.

All apnoea should be classified into one of the following three types based on their pattern of inspiratory effort:

- obstructive apnoea - the inspiratory effort is present throughout the event, i.e. the tape moves, regardless of whether it decreases or increases (figure 5);
- central apnoea - the inspiratory effort is absent throughout the event, i.e. the band does not move (figure 6);
- mixed apnoea - the inspiratory effort is absent in the first part of the apnoea and present in the second part, in other words, the first part is central, and the second is obstructive (figure 6).

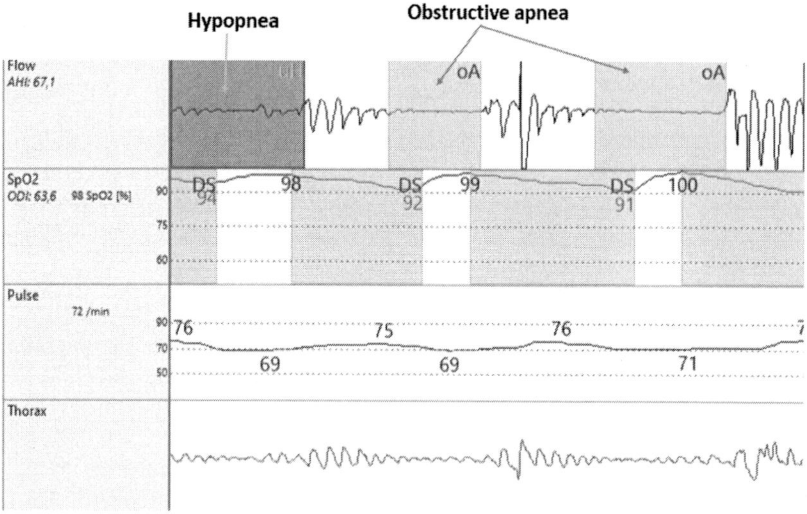

Figure 5. Obstructive Apnoea [Photo Source: Personal Archive]

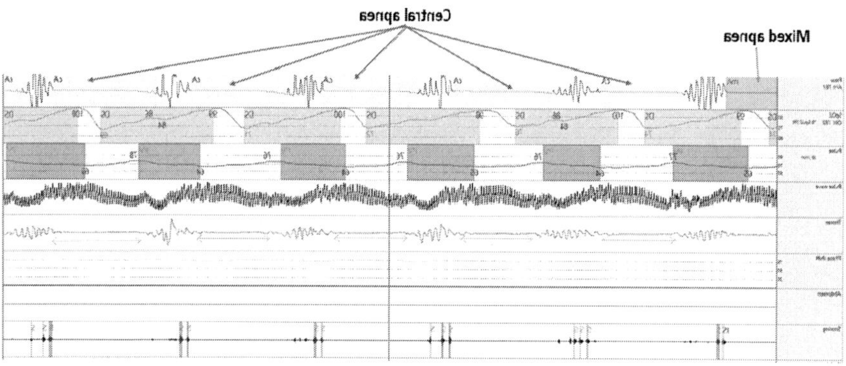

Figure 6. Central Apnoea [Photo Source: Personal Archive]

The advantages of sleep polygraph are:

- it can be performed on an outpatient basis, without requiring a specialized laboratory;
- does not require night surveillance personnel;
- the patient's stress is lower because he is not equipped with EEG electrodes and can sleep at home;

- it is less expensive;
- allows periodic control of the effectiveness of continuous positive airway pressure treatment.

The major disadvantage of the method is the lack of EEG and the certainty that the patient is asleep at certain moments of the recording. However, for severe cases, with suggestive clinical symptoms and a high probability of Pickwick syndrome (obese and sleepy patients), polygraph is a simple and effective diagnostic method.

When the patient does not fit into the classic type of the disease, and the recording marks a relatively small number of apnoea/hypopnea per hour of sleep (Apnoea-hypopnea index = 5-10/hour), referral to a polysomnography laboratory is necessary to confirm the diagnosis [9, 10].

In conclusion, despite its limitations, respiratory polygraph is a very important tool for determining diagnostic algorithms for obstructive sleep apnoea syndrome. This is much more accessible than polysomnography and is based on rules for correcting sleep tracks that are clear and standardized. For this reason, we believe it will be increasingly used by all respiratory health professionals.

References

1. Lyons MM, Bhatt NY, Pack AI, et al. Global burden of sleep-disordered breathing and its implications. Respirology. 2020; 25:690–702.
2. Locke B, Lee J, Sundar K. OSA and Chronic Respiratory Disease: Mechanisms and Epidemiology. Int J Environ Res Public Health. 2022 May; 19(9): 5473.
3. Munteanu I. Guidelines for the management of adult patients with respiratory disorders during sleep. Bucharest: Romanian Society of Pneumology; 2024.\
4. American Academy of Sleep Medicine. International classification of sleep disorders. 3a. ed. Darien, IL: American Academy of Sleep Medicine; 2014.\
5. Platon AL, Stelea CG, Boisteanu O, et al. An Update on Obstructive Sleep Apnea Syndrome—A Literature Review. Medicina (Kaunas). 2023 Aug; 59(8):1459.
6. Chiner Em Canovas C, Molina V, et al. Home Respiratory Polygraphy is Useful in the Diagnosis of Childhood Obstructive Sleep Apnea Syndrome. J Clin Med. 2020 Jul; 9(7): 2067.

7. Collop NA, Anderson WM, Boehlecke B, et al. Clinical guidelines for the use of unattended portable monitors in the diagnosis of obstructive sleep apnea in adult patients. Portable Monitoring Task Force of the American Academy of Sleep Medicine. J Clin Sleep Med. 2007; 3(7):737-747.
8. Berry RB, Quan SF, Abreu AR, et al; for the American Academy of Sleep Medicine. The AASM Manual for the Scoring of Sleep and Associated Events: Rules, Terminology and Technical Specifications, Version 2.6. Darien, IL: American Academy of Sleep Medicine; 2020.
9. Corra-Penafiel J, Barbe F, Pepin JL. Ambulatory monitoring in the diagnosis and management of obstructive sleep apnoea syndrome. European Respiratory Review 2013 22: 312-324.
10. Candela A, Hernandez L, Asensio S, et al. Validation of a respiratory polygraphy system in the diagnosis of sleep apnea syndrome. Arch Bronconeumol. 2005 Feb;41(2):71-7.

CHAPTER 9

CRITERIA FOR DISABILITY IN OPHTHALMOLOGY

SUHER ABDURAMAN AND IOANA SOARE

Medical criteria are used by all insurance companies (both state and private/ pension funds or life insurers) to limit access to disability pension/benefit. Thus, only medium and severely affected patients have access to some insurance benefits.

Disability in ophthalmology refers to visual impairments that significantly impact an individual's ability to perform essential daily tasks, even with optimal correction such as glasses, contact lenses, or surgery. These impairments can range from mild to severe and may include conditions like reduced visual acuity, narrowing of the visual field, or complete blindness [1]. Factors such as the inability to read, recognize faces, navigate safely, or drive are common indicators of visual disability. Legal definitions and thresholds for disability often vary by region, but they generally involve specific criteria for visual acuity and field loss. Ophthalmological disabilities can arise from congenital conditions, diseases like glaucoma or macular degeneration, injuries, or age-related changes, enhancing the importance of the early diagnosis and the constant intervention to improve the quality of life.

In Romania, the criteria for determining the functional deficit in ophthalmology are established by Order No 1243 bis of 2022. The assessment is based on two main parameters: visual acuity and the visual field of the better eye, with optimal correction. Visual acuity measures central vision (using an optotype) and is assessed both with and without corrective lenses. The evaluation considers the better eye with the most effective correction. The visual field measures peripheral vision and is evaluated using a Goldman perimeter (manual) or a computerized device, with results expressed as the degree of peripheral reduction. For an accurate assessment of visual function, additional objective tests are recommended based on the diagnosis. These include corneal topography for corneal conditions like keratoconus, ultrasound for issues involving transparent media such as the lens or vitreous, angiography (AFG), photography, and electroretinography (ERG) for vascular, degenerative, or hereditary retinal conditions, and optical coherence tomography (OCT) or visual evoked potentials (VEP) for optic nerve damage.

Persons with disabilities (currently referred to as individuals with special needs) may be entitled to income as a substitute for wages (disability pension for those with work experience), disability allowance (special needs allowance), and related rights. Patients with ophthalmological conditions are eligible for both a disability certificate and a disability pension, depending on the criteria in force (Romania).

In ophthalmology, the criteria for assessing disability are primarily based on visual acuity and visual field measurements. These criteria help classify the severity of a visual impairment and are essential for determining the level of functional limitation and the need for social and medical support (Table 1). As the population ages and the prevalence of conditions like macular degeneration, glaucoma, and diabetic retinopathy increases, understanding and applying these criteria will become even more important. Additionally, these clinical assessments are crucial not only for medical diagnosis but also for ensuring that individuals with visual impairments receive the appropriate legal protections, financial support, and accommodations to lead independent and fulfilling lives.

Parameters	Functional deficit	Work capacity	Degree of disability
• visual acuity (VA) of 1/2 to 1/3 (0.5–0.3) in the better eye with correction • a peripheral visual field (VF) reduced by 5° to a maximum of 10° In cases of monocular vision, VA is 1 without correction, with a normal VF.	Mild 20-49%	Preserved Slight limitation of activity	No
• VA between 1/4 and 1/10 (0.25–0.10) in the better eye with correction	Moderate 50-69%	Lost at least halfway of work capacity,	Grade III

• a VF reduced by 10 to 20° For monocular vision, VA ranges from less than 1 to 2/3, 1/2, or 1/3 with permanent correction and a normal VF. Visual evoked potentials (VEP) and electroretinography (ERG) remain normal.		moderate limitation of activity	
• VA ranging from 1/12 (0.08) to 1/20 (0.05) with correction in the better eye • a VF reduced by 20° to 40° Retinal function is diminished but still partially functional, as indicated by altered VEP. Monocular VA is less than 1/3 to 1/9, with a VF reduction of 10° to 20°.	Severe 70-89%	Work capacity limitated	Grade II
• VA between 1/25 and 1/50 (0.04–0.02) in the better eye with correction, or the inability to perceive light or hand movement. • Concentric VF reduction is equal to or less than 20°, resembling a "tunnel vision" effect. Monocular VA is less than or equal to 1/10 with permanent correction, and VF is reduced to 20-30°.	Profound 90-100%	Work and self-care capacity limitated	Grade I

Table 1. Functional Deficiency Criteria in Romania

Terms in the USA - blind versus visually impaired [5]. You're considered blind if the vision in your better eye, using a correcting lens, is 20/200 (nb1/10) or less, or if your visual field is 20° or less in your better eye [6].

"If your vision doesn't meet our definition of blindness, you may still qualify for disability benefits," the SSA says. "This is true if your vision problems alone, or combined with other health problems, prevent you from working" [6].

In Germany they use criteria for visually impaired patients - less than 1/10 visual acuity and less than 10°visual field in the better eye [7].

References

1. https://www.ncoa.org/article/what-is-considered-a-disability-by-social-security/
2. Ioana Soare. Criterii de pensionare in oftalmologie. Viata Medicala; 2019
   https://www.viata-medicala.ro/criterii-de-pensionare-in-oftalmologie-18180
3. Monitorul Oficial al României. Partea I, Nr 1243 bis/22.XII.2022
4. https://www.euroblind.org/convention/article-7/romania
5. https://www.ncoa.org/article/what-is-considered-a-disability-by-social-security/
6. Social Security Administration. If You're Blind or Have Low Vision – How We Can Help. 2023. Found on the internet at https://www.ssa.gov/pubs/EN-05-10052.pdf
7. https://www.bmas.de/DE/Soziales/Soziale-Entschaedigung/Rundschreiben/Anhaltspunkte-aerztliche-Gutachtertaetigkeit.html

PART 5

ERRORS

CHAPTER 1

ECG TRACE RECORDING ARTIFACTS

GABRIELA SILVIA GHEORGHE

The electrocardiogram ECG represents the recording of the electrical potential differences between 2 points on the body surface, differences that change depending on the electrical activity of the heart [1].

The appearance of recorded deflections depends on several factors:

- the correctness of the recording (the placement of the electrodes/leads, the paper speed and the amplitude of the signal;
- the surrounding tissues (fat, muscles), with low conductivity, decreasing the amplitude of the vectors.
- the filtering mechanism of parasitic signals.

A. Calibrating the machine - Paper scroll speed is generally 25mm/sec. At this speed, a time interval of 0.04 sec elapses between 2 thin vertical lines and 0.2 sec between 2 thick lines. If lower speeds are used (10 mm/sec) the time between two thin vertical lines is 0.01 sec, the QRS complexes are narrower, the intervals are seemingly shorter and the heart rate is apparently fast. At the paper scrolling speed of (50 mm/sec) the elapsed time between two thin vertical lines is 0.02 sec. The QRS complexes are wider, mimicking bundle branch blocks, the intervals are apparently longer, and the heart rate is apparently slower.

B. Wave amplitude calibration is done following the 10 mm=1 mV rule. The ascent of the waves from the isoelectric line to the maximum level must be done in no more than 0.01-0.02 sec. Registration errors may occur (fig.1):

- Overshooting= overestimation of the size of the deflections, when the standard registers a peak on the upward slope (instead of being rectangular);
- Overdamping= underestimation of the size of the waves, when the standard is with rounded corners.

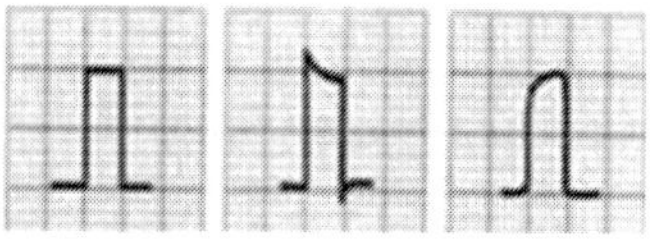

Fig 1. Normal calibration (left), overshooting (middle), overdamping (right)

C. Correct electrode placement is essential for correct interpretation of ECGs. For example, reversal of the electrode attached to the right arm with the one attached to the left arm can create the false image of myocardial infarction (fig.2, fig.3) [2].

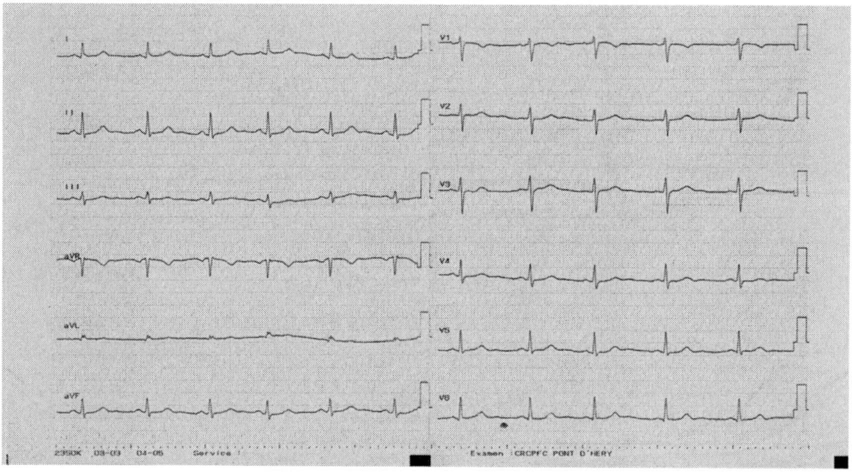

Fig 2. ECG recorded with electrodes placed in the correct position G.S. Gheorghe Archive

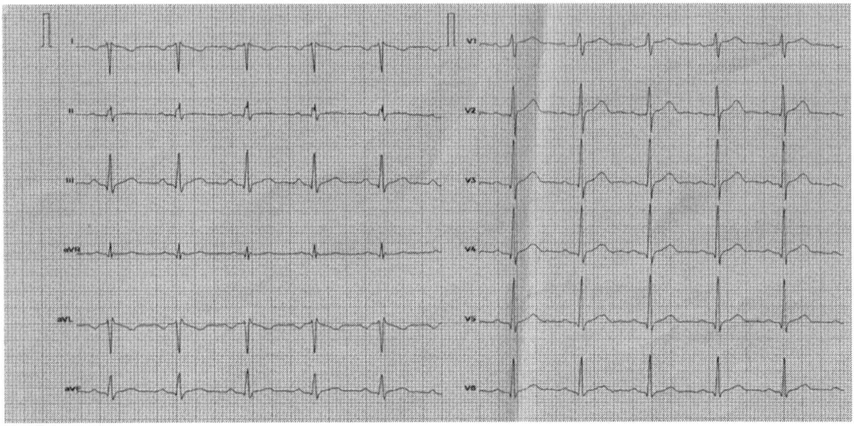

Fig.3 False infarct image (predominantly negative QRS complex in D1, aVL) by inverting the electrode on the right arm with the one on the left arm G.S. Gheorghe Archive

D. The influence of the surrounding tissues, which attenuate the intensity of the electrical signal of the heart.

- Low voltage occurs in obesity, large breasts, pulmonary hyperinflation, pericardial effusion or left pleural effusion. In these situations, ventricular hypertrophy is underdiagnosed on the ECG.
- Young, thin patients may have wider QRS complexes, mimicking ventricular hypertrophy.

E. Interpretation errors can also occur due to the association of several cardiac pathologies, by the cancellation of electrical vectors.

Conclusion

ECG interpretation must always be done in the clinical context.

References

1. Dale Dubin, Rapid Interpretation of EKG's (6th ed.), Medical Publishing House, Bucharest, 2024
2. García-Niebla J, Llontop-García P, Valle-Racero JI, Serra-Autonell G, Batchvarov VN, de Luna AB. Technical mistakes during the acquisition of the electrocardiogram. Ann Noninvasive Electrocardiol.

2009 Oct;14(4):389-403. doi: 10.1111/j.1542-474X.2009.00328.x. PMID: 19804517; PMCID: PMC6932211.

CHAPTER 2

ERRORS AND LABORATORY MEDICINE – CAUSES AND STRATEGIES

MANOLE COJOCARU

Medical errors negatively impact the patient, the family, the clinicians, the support staff and the healthcare facility. The term 'error' is used in the medical articles in general and should be employed for errors in laboratory medicine.

These patient samples measurements are a central part of modern clinical management, they are used by clinicians to diagnose disease phases, to guide treatment course and to determine prognosis.

The preanalytical phase has a significant impact on the quality of laboratory results. Articles mention that pre- and post-analytical steps of the total testing process are more error-prone, id est outside of the laboratory. A precise test will produce similar results when the test is repeated multiple times. Accuracy (or rather trueness) is a measure of the proximity of the test results to the true value. Precision measures reliability and reproducibility. Bias or systematic error is a form of measurement error that skews the results to one side.

Laboratory errors often occur outside the laboratory, as medical testing and procedures are performed by individuals with various levels of quality control training. Laboratory analyses are crucial for diagnosis, follow-up and treatment decisions [1]. Measurements in laboratory medicine have a degree of uncertainty. This uncertainty is often called error and refers to imprecisions and inaccuracies in measurement, as the difference between the true value of the measured sample and the measured value.

One of the types of error is the systematic error, also called bias, because these errors are reproducible and skew the results consistently in the same direction. Regulation of quality in the health care sector is based on accreditation, certification, quality monitoring, patient's rights, standard operation processes and standards of health care quality [2].

Efforts have been made in the last years, in the comprehension and the reduction of the errors in medicine [3].

The errors in the laboratory medicine are named also mistakes, blunders, defects, outliers, unacceptable results, quality failure.

Minimizing uncertainty in the laboratory diagnostics should be made by implementing a Total Quality Management system.

Clinical laboratories have long focused their attention on quality control methods and quality assessment programs dealing with analytical aspects of testing [4].

The error rates in the laboratory activities are far lower than those seen in clinical health care.

Errors in laboratory medicine are part of a much wider issue, commonly known as "diagnostic error".

In fact, over the past decades, a ten-fold reduction in the analytical error rate has been achieved thanks to improvements in the reliability and the standardization of analytical techniques, reagents and instrumentation.

Advances in information technology, quality control and quality assurance methods have made a valuable contribution to error reduction. Patient identification should be performed by asking open questions and/or comparing the patient's identification (barcoded) bracelet using at least two identifiers. Collection tubes should be labelled directly before or after phlebotomy, but always in the presence of the patient.

However, although the state-of-the-art highlights that pre-analytical then post-analytical phases are more vulnerable to errors [5].

The laboratory work might be divided into 3 phases (pre-analytical, analytical and post-analytical). The accurate identification of the patient and the appropriate labelling of blood collection tubes are crucial steps for preventing diagnostic errors and mismanagement of patient data.

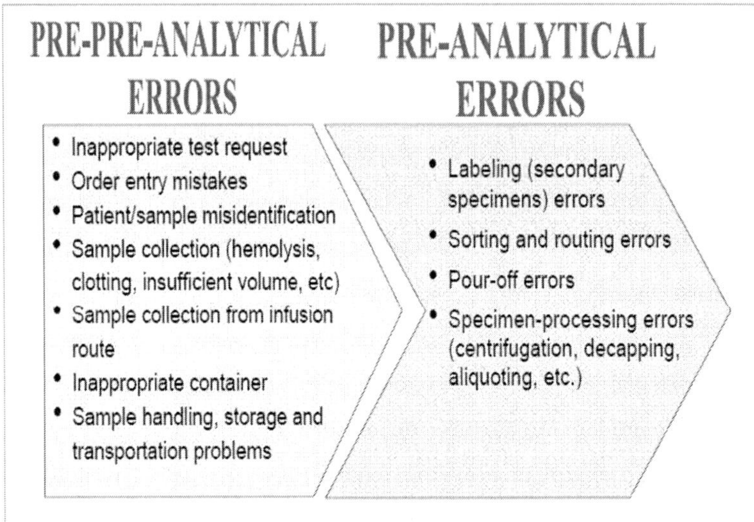

Figure 1 [1]

Identification errors of a patient or a specimen has the potential to cause patients harm. Pre-analytical errors or more accurately pre-pre-analytical errors are estimated to account for up to 70% of all mistakes made in laboratory diagnostics, most of which arise from problems in patient preparation and sample collection, transportation, preparation for analysis and storage.

Pre-analytical errors can occur at the time of patient assessment, test order entry, request completion, patient identification, specimen collection, specimen transport or specimen receipt in the laboratory.

Written procedures must be implemented.

Visual detection of hemolysis must be abandoned, but new samples should be examined [6].

There is still evidence indicating that analytical quality remains a major issue, documented for immunoassays [7].

The issue of analytical interference does not only affect immunoassays. As an example, monoclonal proteins may affect some analyses (glucose, bilirubin, C-reactive protein, creatinine and albumin).

To mention only a few examples, the specimen may be drawn from the wrong patient; erroneous low calcium and alkaline phosphatase may be misinterpreted, when potassium-ethylene-diamine-tetra-acetic acid (potassium-EDTA) contamination is not identified; pseudo-hyperkalemia due to extreme leukocytosis may lead to unnecessary and even potentially dangerous treatment. Collecting blood in a non-fasted state and even chewing of a sugar-free gum may influence laboratory parameters. Moreover, the concentration of specific analytes, e.g. catecholamines, may be influenced by the type of aliments ingested recently.

Information on physical activity, as well as intake of drugs (time, dosage), are also important for the accurate interpretation of test results. Moreover, patients should rest for at least 15 minutes, either lying or sitting before blood collection [8]. In special cases, e.g. catecholamines in plasma, these demands may be even more stringent. Blood samples should be collected in the morning, to prevent the impact of diurnal variation. The time of sample collection should always be documented, to verify whether laboratory analyses are performed within the time of stability of the respective parameter. Nevertheless, the information about the preparation of the patient should be documented to avoid misinterpretation of results [9]. Blood should never be drawn at the infusion site or proximal thereof. In case intravenous lines cannot be avoided for blood collection, the flushing of the line and the subsequent discard of a certain blood volume should be carried out correctly. If venous stasis cannot be avoided, the tourniquet should be released within one minute while the blood is collected into the first tube to avoid alterations due to fluid shifts. Collecting blood in the appropriate tubes and in the correct order of draw is crucial to avoid additive carryover. Potassium-EDTA contamination of heparin samples may result in spurious hyperkalemia and low concentrations of calcium due to EDTA sequestration. Tubes need to be filled up to the indicated volume, inverted once immediately after blood collection and at least five to ten times, as indicated by manufacturers, at the end of the phlebotomy procedure. This practice will prevent rejection of specimen due to clotting. Especially for coagulation assays, correct filling of tubes is essential to ensure an adequate blood/citrate-ratio. The analytical stability of analytes is highly dependent on the time passed between blood collection and analysis, as well as on temperature and other ambient conditions (i.e. light exposure). Whereas some parameters may be stable for a long time, others may already be altered one hour after blood collection or even earlier. To ensure the right sample transportation, local requirements have to be defined and distributed to all clinicians, nursing staff and carriers. A survey among European laboratories on preanalytical practices for coagulation tests recently found that only 42% of participating laboratories are actually monitoring temperature during transportation. Haemolysis, icterus and lipemia may lead to erroneous test results of several analytes due to physical and chemical interferences [10].

The lack of inter-changeability between different methods and clinical laboratories is not considered an "analytical error".

In the post-analytical phase, the clinician interprets the results and makes decisions accordingly.

Diagnostic errors might be defined as unintentionally delayed (sufficient information was available earlier), wrong (another diagnosis made before the correct one) or missed (no diagnosis made).

Pragmatically, error prevention, error detection and error management are part of the Total Quality Management system [10].

Medical laboratory professionals and physicians must "understand their mutual ownership and work together to ensure that patients are safer" [11].

Conclusion

The Evidence Based Medicine and the Total Quality Management system can help reducing errors in laboratory medicine.

Defining pre- and post-analytical steps as error - prone should increase the importance to implement targeted procedures.

References

1. Plebani M, Diagnostic Errors and Laboratory Medicine – Causes and Strategies. EJIFCC. 2015; 26(1): 7-14.
2. Hammerling JA, A Review of Medical Errors in Laboratory Diagnostics and Where We Are Today. Laboratory Medicine, 2012; 43: 41-4.
3. Mario Plebani The detection and prevention of errors in laboratory medicine. Ann Clin Biochem. 2010; 47(Pt 2): 101-10.
4. Howanitz PJ. Errors in laboratory medicine: Practical lessons to improve patient safety. Archives of Pathology and Laboratory Medicine. 2005; 129(10): 1252-61.

5. Mrazek C, Lippi G, Keppel MH, et al. Errors within the total laboratory testing process, from test selection to medical decision-making - A review of causes, consequences, surveillance and solutions. Biochem Med (Zagreb). 2020; 30(2): 020502.
6. Dikmen ZG, Pinar A, Akbiyik F. Specimen rejection in laboratory medicine: Necessary for patient safety? Biochem Med (Zagreb). 2015; 25: 377-85.
7. Kalra J. Medical errors: impact on clinical laboratories and other critical areas. Clin Biochem. 2004; 37(12): 1052-62.
8. Valenstein PN, Sirota RL Identification errors in pathology and laboratory medicine. Clin Lab Med. 2004; 24(4): 979-96.
9. Plebani M Errors in clinical laboratories or errors in laboratory medicine? Clinical Chemistry and Laboratory Medicine 2006; 44(6): 750-9
10. Miligy DA Laboratory errors and patient safety. Int J Health Care Qual Assur. 2015; 28(1): 2-10.
11. Soare Ioana, Explained Medical Analyses, 9th edition, Etna Publishing House, Bucharest, Romania, 2020, pg. 195-202

CHAPTER 3

ERRORS IN SPIROMETRY – INSURANCE MEDICINE

CONSTANTIN GHIMUȘ
AND PARASCHIVA POSTOLACHE

The spirometry is an method for the evaluation of the respiratory function. It is used in the diagnosis and monitoring of the obstructive and the restrictive lung diseases. However, the quality and the accuracy of the spirometry tests can be influenced by numerous factors, which can lead to significant errors. In order to obtain accurate and reliable results, it is crucial that every step of the testing process is done correctly. Errors in patient preparation, technique execution, equipment maintenance, and data interpretation can lead to misdiagnosis and inappropriate therapeutic decisions. By implementing standardized procedures, continuous staff training, use of advanced technology, and rigorous performance monitoring, these errors can be significantly reduced, thereby improving the quality of patient care [1].

I. Pre-analytical errors

1. Patient preparation

One of the most common sources of error in spirometry is inadequate patient preparation. According to the guidelines, patients should avoid smoking, drinking alcohol and vigorous exercise at least one hour before the test. Also, the use of certain bronchodilator drugs should be stopped before the test, according to the doctor's recommendations [2].

- smoking can temporarily affect lung function, resulting in falsely low values of FEV1 and FVC;

- drinking alcohol and coffee before the spirometry: the alcohol can depress the respiratory system, while the coffee, due to its caffeine content, can have temporary bronchodilator effects [3];
- intense physical exercises can affect the lung function by inducing bronchoconstriction or muscle fatigue;
- the use of bronchodilators: the short-acting drugs should be avoided 4-6 hours before, and the long-acting drugs 12-24 hours before the test [4].

The environmental conditions such as temperature and humidity can affect the spirometry measurements. The spirometry equipment is sensitive to these variables, and results can be inaccurate, if the test is performed under inappropriate conditions. It is essential that the test is performed in a controlled environment with stable temperature and humidity [5].

2. Ineffective instructions

Inadequate training of the patient on the blowing technique can lead to erroneous results. It is essential that the medical staff provide clear instructions and demonstrate the correct technique, ensuring that the patient understands and can perform the maneuver correctly. Lack of proper training can lead to errors in technique, such as insufficient or uneven blowing, affecting test results. Anxiety and discomfort can also influence the patient's performance during the test. Creating a calm environment and providing reassurance and detailed explanations can help reduce anxiety and improve patient cooperation [6].

3. Equipment calibration and test protocol compliance

Inadequate or improper spirometer calibration is a common pre-analytical error. Equipment must be calibrated daily to ensure measurement accuracy. The use of standardized calibration syringes is essential to maintain the accuracy of the equipment.

Failure to follow the standardized testing protocol may result in inconsistent results. It is important that all spirometry tests follow a clear protocol, including equipment check procedures and breathing techniques [7].

4. Poor verification of the patient's health

The health of the patient on the day of the test can influence the results. For example, a respiratory infection can affect the lung function temporarily. It is essential that doctors assess the patient's health and decide if rescheduling the test is necessary [8].

II. Analytical errors

1. Non-compliant equipment

The calibration and the maintenance of the spirometry equipment are critical to obtaining accurate results. The spirometers should be calibrated daily, using a standardized calibration syringe. Uncalibrated or defective equipment can introduce significant errors in the measurements of the respiratory flows and volumes [9].

2. Operator variability

The skill and experience of the operator are determining factors in obtaining correct spirometry results. Operators must be well trained and follow strict testing protocols to minimize inter- and intra-operator variability. One study showed that errors introduced by operators can vary significantly, influencing the accuracy of diagnoses [10].

3. Inadequate breathing technique

Insufficient expiration - One of the most common errors is inadequate expiration. To obtain accurate measurements, the patient must exhale completely and with maximum force. Incomplete expiration or lack of force can lead to underestimation of FEV1 and FVC.

Incomplete inspiration - Equally important is the timing of inspiration. If the patient does not fully inhale before exhaling, the measured air volume will be inaccurate. It is essential that the patient inhale to full lung capacity before forced expiration.

Interrupted expiration - Interruptions in airflow during expiration can distort results. These can be caused by coughing, changing the position of the mouth on the mouthpiece, or other factors that disrupt the continuous flow of air [11].

4. Incorrect body position

Upright position - The patient should sit upright with the trunk straight to ensure full lung expansion. Incorrect posture can limit lung capacity and lead to inaccurate results.

Mouthpiece Support - The patient should hold the mouthpiece firmly but comfortably to prevent air leakage. Any leakage can affect the measurements and lead to erroneous interpretations [12].

5. Patient cooperation and effort

Lack of maximal effort - Spirometry requires maximal effort from the patient to obtain accurate measurements. A suboptimal effort can lead to an underestimation of lung function. Appropriate training and encouragement of the patient are essential to ensure adequate effort.

Anxiety and distrust - Anxiety or distrust can influence the patient's performance. Patients should be informed and reassured about the spirometry procedure to reduce their anxiety and improve cooperation [13].

6. Technical problems and equipment handling

Air leakage - Any air leakage around the mouthpiece or nose can affect the measurements. It is important that the patient uses a nose clip and holds the mouthpiece tightly to prevent leakage.

Motion artifacts - Sudden movements of the patient or mouthpiece can create artifacts in the spirometry data. The patient must remain still during the test to avoid these problems [14].

7. Data interpretation and validation

Lack of reproducibility - To ensure the validity of the results, it is essential that the maneuver is repeated several times and the measurements are reproducible. Large differences between repetitions may indicate inadequate technique or inconsistent effort.

Acceptability of Measurements - The ATS/ERS Guidelines specify clear criteria for the acceptability of spirometry measurements. These criteria include no air leaks, continuous maximal expiration for at least 6 seconds, and a smooth flow-volume curve. Any deviation from these criteria may invalidate the results [15].

III. Post-analytical errors

1. Incorrect interpretation of results

Lack of familiarity with guidelines - one of the most common post-analytical errors is the incorrect interpretation of results due to ignorance or failure to follow current guidelines, such as those of the American Thoracic Society (ATS) and the European Respiratory Society (ERS). These guidelines provide clear criteria for the interpretation of spirometry results, including reference values, criteria for acceptability and reproducibility.

Factors such as the patient's age, sex, height, weight, and ethnicity must be considered when interpreting spirometric results. Ignoring these variables can lead to erroneous interpretations. For example, normal values for FEV1 and FVC vary significantly by these demographic characteristics [16].

2. Error in data calculation and reporting

Mathematical errors in the calculation of spirometry parameters, such as the FEV1/FVC ratio, can lead to wrong conclusions. Using the right software and double-checking your calculations is essential to avoid these errors. Incomplete reporting of data or inclusion of incorrect information may compromise subsequent clinical evaluation. All relevant measurements and observations should be included in the report, and the data should be checked for accuracy before being forwarded to the physician [17].

3. Problems related to the validation and verification of the results

A crucial aspect of spirometry is ensuring reproducibility of results. Failure to repeat tests to verify consistency of measurements can lead to unreliable results. The guidelines recommend that at least three acceptable maneuvers and two reproducible measurements be obtained for test validation. Accepting results that do not meet the quality criteria can lead to erroneous interpretations. Results must meet the acceptability criteria established by the ATS/ERS, which include no air leaks, a smooth flow-volume curve, and continuous maximal expiration for at least 6 seconds [6].

4. Inadequate communication of results

Spirometry results should be communicated clearly and concisely. Ambiguous or incomplete language in reports can create confusion and affect clinical decisions. Using a standardized reporting format can help avoid these problems. Delay in reporting results may affect patient management. The spirometry results must be sent promptly to the doctor in charge to allow rapid therapeutic decisions [18].

5. Problems with automatic interpretation

The use of automated software to interpret spirometry results can lead to errors if the results are not checked manually. Software can help identify trends and anomalies, but the final interpretation should be made by an experienced specialist. The software algorithms may have limitations in interpreting the complex or atypical cases. It is important for the clinicians to consider them in interpreting the results [19].

Impact of the errors

The misdiagnosis of obstructive lung diseases can lead to inappropriate or unnecessary treatments. In addition, errors can affect the monitoring of disease progression and the evaluation of the response to treatment, leading to wrong clinical decisions [20].

How to reduce errors

1. Standardization of procedures

Implementing and following standardized guidelines for performing spirometry can significantly reduce errors. Organizations such as the American Thoracic Society (ATS) and the European Respiratory Society (ERS) have published detailed guidelines on correct spirometry procedures [2].

2. Continuous staff training

Ongoing training of medical staff in spirometry techniques and data interpretation is essential to maintain proficiency and reduce errors. Periodic certification and recertification programs can help ensure a high level of expertise, ensuring operator competence, reducing variability and user-introduced errors [21].

3. Use of advanced technology

The use of modern, well-maintained equipment can reduce technical errors and improve the accuracy of measurements. Advanced digital spirometers can provide real-time feedback, helping to identify and correct performance errors as they occur. Data interpretation software can also improve the accuracy of analyses and alert operators to abnormal values. Following the guidelines for calibrating and maintaining spirometry equipment is essential to obtaining accurate results [3].

4. Performance monitoring and evaluation

Regular monitoring and evaluation of the medical team's performance can help identify and correct errors. These processes involve regularly reviewing spirometry results and comparing them to established standards, as well as assessing the skills of operators [22].

5. Multidisciplinary evaluation

Decisions about work ability and retirement should be made by multidisciplinary teams that include pulmonologists, occupational physicians, insurance medical expers and others. This can help to correctly interpret spirometry results and take into account all factors relevant to the patient's health and work capacity [8].

6. Continuous monitoring of patients

Regular assessment of lung function can help identify any changes in the patient's health early. Continuous monitoring allows adjustment of treatment plans and decisions about work capacity, ensuring that patients receive the right care at the right time [6].

Impact of spirometry errors on work ability

Spirometry plays a crucial role not only in the diagnosis and treatment of respiratory diseases, but also in the evaluation of patients' work capacity. Spirometry errors can have a significant impact on work capacity and retirement decisions, directly influencing patients' professional and financial lives.

IV. The impact of errors on work capacity

1. Underestimation of the severity of the disease

If spirometry results do not accurately reflect the degree of pulmonary obstruction or restriction, patients may be considered able/fit to continue their work, despite the fact that their health may prevent them from performing their work duties effectively. This can lead to:

- Low performance at work: patients with underestimated respiratory problems may have difficulty maintaining an adequate level of performance, affecting their productivity and quality of work;
- Increasing the risk of work accidents by fatigue and breathing difficulties, mostly in dangerous work environments;
- Absenteeism: underdiagnosed patients may have frequent episodes of disease exacerbations, leading to frequent short term sick leave or plain absences, and career instability [20].

2. Overestimation of the severity of the disease

Patients may be considered unfit for work and thus excluded from professional activity unjustifiably. This can lead to:

- Loss of income: the inability to work can seriously affect the financial situation of patients and their families;
- Psychological impact: forced retirement or job loss can lead to depression, anxiety and low self-esteem;
- Social isolation: not having a job can lead to social isolation and the loss of daily interactions that are essential for psychological well-being [23].

V. Disability criteria based on spirometry

Spirometry, a non-invasive pulmonary function test, can influence insurance medicine evaluations, especially in cases where an individual's work capacity is compromised by a respiratory condition. Respiratory diseases and their impact on work capacity

b) Chronic obstructive pulmonary disease (COPD) -. The significant reduction of the FEV1 and FVC may indicate a reduced work capacity.
c) Bronchial asthma - can limit the work capacity due to the recurrent episodes of bronchoconstriction. Spirometry is used to monitor lung function and assess disease control. Low FEV1 values and the FEV1/FVC ratio may indicate uncontrolled asthma, affecting the retirement decision.
d) Pulmonary fibrosis - progressive disease characterized by scarring of lung tissue, which leads to breathing difficulties. Spirometry can help assess the severity of lung damage by measuring forced vital

capacity (FVC). Reduced FVC may reflect reduced lung capacity, influencing work capacity and, implicitly, the decision to retire.

e) Occupational lung diseases - occupational exposure to harmful substances such as silica dust, asbestos or metal fumes can lead to lung diseases such as silicosis or asbestosis. Spirometry is used to monitor the lung function of exposed workers and to assess the need for early retirement due to respiratory impairment [16].

In many countries, the assessment of lung function by spirometry is an important criterion for the award of sickness pension. For example, patients with severe COPD may be eligible for early retirement if their lung function is below a certain threshold. Spirometric values used in these assessments include:

- Maximum FEV1: evaluates the severity of the obstructive disease. An FEV1< 40% of the predicted value is used as one of the criteria for the disability;
- FEV1/FVC (Forced Vital Capacity) ratio: A low ratio indicates severe obstruction, and values below 0.7 are frequently used to diagnose and evaluate COPD [17].

VI. The impact of errors on retirement decisions

Spirometry provides objective measurements of lung function, essential for assessing work capacity. Parameters such as FEV1, FVC and the FEV1/FVC ratio are used to determine the severity of respiratory diseases and to assess their impact on daily activities and work capacity.

In many countries, early retirement decisions on medical grounds are based on strict criteria, which include assessment of lung function. Spirometry plays a critical role in determining eligibility for early retirement by providing objective data to support or disprove the need for retirement. At the same time, this technique is used to monitor the evolution of respiratory diseases and to evaluate the effectiveness of treatment. Changes in lung function over time may influence decisions to reassess work capacity and may warrant revision of the retirement decision.

Errors that lead to underestimation of the severity of respiratory disease can result in a patient being considered fit for work, even though their work capacity is compromised. This can lead to continuing work in inadequate conditions, adversely affecting the patient's health and increasing the risk of complications [24].

Similarly, errors that lead to overestimation of disease severity can lead to unwarranted early retirement, which can have important economic and social implications for the patient. Unjustified retirement can affect the patient's self-esteem and lead to the loss of necessary income.

References

1. American Thoracic Society. Standardization of Spirometry 1994 Update. Am J Respir Crit Care Med. 2005;152(3):766-779. doi:10.1164/ajrccm.152.3.766.
2. Miller MR, Hankinson J, Brusasco V, et al. Standardization of spirometry. Eur Respir J. 2005;26(2):319-338. doi:10.1183/09031936.05.00034805.
3. Pellegrino R, Viegi G, Brusasco V, et al. Interpretative strategies for lung function tests. Eur Respir J. 2005;26(5):948-968. doi:10.1183/09031936.05.00035205.
4. Enright PL. Office spirometry: a practical guide to the selection and use of spirometers. Respir Care. 2003;48(8):773-786. doi:10.4187/respcare.48.8.773.
5. Quanjer PH, Stanojevic S, Cole TJ, et al. Multi-ethnic reference values for spirometry for the 3–95-yr age range: the global lung function 2012 equations. Eur Respir J. 2012;40(6):1324-1343. doi:10.1183/09031936.00080312.
6. Hankinson JL, Odencrantz JR, Fedan KB. Spirometric reference values from a sample of the general U.S. population. Am J Respir Crit Care Med. 1999;159(1):179-187. doi:10.1164/ajrccm.159.1.9712108.
7. Crapo RO, Morris AH, Gardner RM. Reference spirometric values using techniques and equipment that meet ATS recommendations. Am Rev Respir Dis. 1981;123(6):659-664. doi:10.1164/arrd.1981.123.6.659.
8. Schermer TR, et al. Evaluation of the short-form 36-item questionnaire to measure health-related quality of life in patients with chronic obstructive pulmonary disease. Br J Gen Pract. 2003;53(492):659-664. doi:10.3399/bjgp03X961282.
9. Ruppel GL. Manual of Pulmonary Function Testing. 10th ed. Elsevier Health Sciences; 2009. doi:10.1016/B978-1-4160-4019-2.00001-1.
10. Townsend MC. Spirometry in the Occupational Setting. J Occup Environ Med. 2011;53(5):569-584. doi:10.1097/JOM.0b013e318230788e.
11. Crapo RO, Casaburi R, Coates AL, et al. ATS/ERS Standardization of Lung Function Testing. Eur Respir J. 2002;26(2):319-338.

doi:10.1183/09031936.02.00270302.
12. O'Donnell CR, et al. Reproducibility of forced expiratory volumes. Chest J. 2005;128(3):1053-1063. doi:10.1378/chest.128.3.1053.
13. Burge PS, Lewis SA. The effects of smoking cessation on respiratory health. Respir Med. 2008;102(11):1491-1500. doi:10.1016/j.rmed.2007.08.004.
14. Brusasco V, Crapo R, Viegi G. ATS/ERS Task Force: Standardization of lung function testing. Eur Respir J. 2005;26(2):319-338. doi:10.1183/09031936.05.00034805.
15. Brusasco V, Crapo R, Viegi G. ATS/ERS Task Force: Interpretative strategies for lung function tests. Eur Respir J. 2005;26(5):948-968. doi:10.1183/09031936.05.00035205.
16. Quanjer PH, Stanojevic S, Cole TJ, et al. Multi-ethnic reference values for spirometry for the 3-95 yr age range: the global lung function 2012 equations. Eur Respir J. 2012;40(6):1324-1343. doi:10.1183/09031936.00080312.
17. Enright PL. The use and abuse of office spirometry. Prim Care Respir J. 2008;17(4):238-243. doi:10.1016/j.rmed.2007.08.004.
18. Ruppel GL. Manual of Pulmonary Function Testing. 10th ed. Mosby Elsevier; 2012. doi:10.1016/B978-0-323-07943-1.00001-5.
19. Townsend MC. Confounders and effect modifiers in pulmonary function tests. Chest. 2011;139(1):154-161. doi:10.1378/chest.09-2687.
20. Crapo RO, Casaburi R, Coates AL, et al. ATS/ERS guidelines for the standardization of lung function testing. Eur Respir J. 2002;26(2):319-338. doi:10.1183/09031936.02.00270302.
21. Enright PL, Brusasco V. The repeatability and reliability of spirometry in clinical trials. Eur Respir J. 2008;32(6):1430-1435. doi:10.1183/09031936.00035208.
22. Quanjer PH, Stocks J, Polgar G, Wise M, Karlberg J, Borsboom G. Compilation of reference values for lung function measurements in children. Eur Respir J. 1989;2(3):184-194. doi:10.1183/09031936.05.00035205.
23. Pellegrino R, Viegi G, Brusasco V. Interpretative strategies for lung function tests. Eur Respir J. 2005;26(5):948-968. doi:10.1183/09031936.05.00035205.
24. Ruppel GL. Manual of Pulmonary Function Testing. 10th ed. Mosby Elsevier; 2009. doi:10.1016/B978-0-323-07943-1.00001-5.

CHAPTER 4

ERRORS IN GENERAL AND ORTHOPEDIC SURGERY

ALEXANDRU-EUGEN NICOLAU
AND IOANA SOARE

Medical errors are a pressing health problem leading to prolonged hospitalization with associated costs, disability and death. Surgical errors (SE) are the most common [1].

As experts of Romanian College of Physicians, we assessed 49 such appeals for SE (2009- 2017), targeting 49 patients and 2 appeals from surgeons.

In this group the average age was 52 years (11-85), 26 were men, 67,35% had comorbidities, 89,79% underwent surgery of which 39,53% in emergency, and 51% died. The patients' conditions were classified as follows: hepatobiliopancreatic 9, gastrointestinal 11, tumors 9, trauma 12, miscellaneous 8. Of the doctors complained, 68.65% were surgeons,9.8% were professors of surgery, the hospitals complained of were county hospitals 49% and university clinics 28.6%. The complaints concerned therapeutic errors 68.6%, diagnostic errors 13.7%, miscommunication 9.8%. In 28.6% of the complaints, we found no adverse events, 42.8% were postoperative complications, 16.3% non-imputable errors and 14.3% mistakes (imputable errors). The latter resulted in 3 deaths and 4 disabilities [2]. According to Reason, there was 1 execution error (technical) and 6 errors concerning knowledge and rule-based mistakes [3]. According to Leape, there were 1 therapeutic error, 3 diagnostic errors, 5 prophylactic errors, with 7 latent system errors [4].

From the expertise of the 49 files with complaints to surgeons, we considered that 28.57% were unfounded, to 40.81% were postoperative complications, EA unpreventable, 30.64% were errors, EA preventable, 16.33% not imputable, but unfortunately 14.28% imputable (mistakes).

Imputable errors occurred in 3 women and 4 men with an average age of 37.3 (11-75) years, resulting in 3 deaths, 3 permanent disabilities and a temporary disability [2].

The orthopedic surgery is also subject to errors. Affecting the skeleton, these problems produce movement disorders. The work capacity may be reduced.

Also frequent are the errors in the plastic surgery and gynecologic surgery. They are less discussed from the point of view of the disability generated.

There is a big problem in "repairing" such errors, both in surgery and in orthopedics. Repairing involves always time, repeated surgical interventions, money from the patient or from the insurance companies. Short term sick leave/medical leave is paid by the insurance companies.

Long-Term Sick Leave/disability benefit/invalidity pension is due to the patient long time before the court decision about the error.

Conclusions

A major problem remains the differentiation between the errors, the adverse events, that can be prevented, and the postoperative complications, that cannot be prevented.

References

1. Turrentine FE, Schenk WG, McMurry TL, Tache-Leon CA, Jones RS. Surgical errors and the relationships of disease, risks, and adverse events. Am J Surg. 2020 Dec;220(6):1572-1578
2. Nicolau Alexandru-Eugen, The expertise of some objections addressed to the College of Doctors from Romania regarding claims of surgical errors, J Surgery, 2024; 20(1): 24-39, DOI: 10.22551/JSURG.2024.01.04
3. Reason J. Understanding adverse events: human factors. Qual Health Care. 1995 Jun;4(2):80-9.
4. Leape LL. Error in medicine. JAMA. 1994;272(23):1851-1857
5. Scott SD, Hirschinger LE, Cox KR, et al. The natural history of recovery for the healthcare provider "second victim" after adverse patient events. Qual Saf Health Care.2009 Oct;18(5):325- 30.
6. Brennan TA, Gawande A, Thomas E, Studdert D. Accidental deaths, saved lives, and improved quality. N Engl J Med. 2005; 353:1405–1409

7. Suliburk JW, Buck QM, Pirko CJ, et al. Analysis of Human Performance Deficiencies Associated With Surgical Adverse Events. JAMA Netw Open. 2019 Jul 3;2(7):e198067.

PART 6

PROBLEMS IN ASSESSMENT

CHAPTER 1

CHRONIC PAIN

IOANA SOARE

Chronic pain, persisting over 3 months, is affecting the individual, from a physical, mental, professional and social point of view, causing a functional deficit. It generates a vicious circle with the involvement of the psychological aspects (anxiety, depression), sleeplessness and the aggravation of the basic problem.

The pain is three-dimensional – sensory-discriminative, affective-motivational and cognitive-evaluative [1]. Any chronic pain is fuzzy, diffuse, imprecise, uncertain, incoherent, not clearly determined, as defined by Araujo and Miyahira [2]. Thus pain is not only generated by nociceptive information in the brain, but also by the cultural aspects of the individual's life experience [2].

It is one of the major causes for the medical consult and for the economic loss - increased medical expenses, lost income, lost productivity, compensation payments and legal charges are some of the repercussions of chronic pain. The most common types are: low back pain, headache, pain in cancer or arthritis [3].

Treede and all proposed for ICD-11 a very good classification, to be found in this reference [4].

The first thing that an insurance medical expert does, in front of a patient with chronic pain, is to evaluate a functional deficit, which expresses the severity of the disorders of the body's functions and the mechanisms by which they occur [5].

As an example, in the case of chest pain secondary to heart diseases, we evaluate the frequency, the intensity (VAS scale), the level of effort at which it occurs, the presence of arrhythmias, heart failure, the response to treatment [5].

Functional impairment is quantifiable, standardized through clinical and functional evaluations [5]. For objectification, a percentage calculation is used, realized by fitting into a grid of criteria and norms, which vary for each insurance company/ health insurance company/ house of pensions.

Conclusion

Chronic pain generates suffering, insomnia, sadness and is a major cause of disability.

References

1. Teodorescu Cristian, LUTS are not caused only by Prostatic Diseases, Medical Life nr 29/15.07.2016, pg 7
2. https://www.researchgate.net/publication/221358782_Tridimensional_fuzzy_pain_assessment; Conference: FUZZ-IEEE 2011, IEEE International Conference on Fuzzy Systems, Taipei, Taiwan, 27-30 June, 2011, Proceedings Araujo Ernesto, Miyahira Susana A. In IEEE International Conference on Fuzzy Systems · June 2011 with 41 Reads DOI: 10.1109/FUZZY.2011.6007639 · Source: DBLP, 25.07. 2016
3. https://www.hopkinsmedicine.org/health/conditions-and-diseases/chronic-pain
4. Treede RD, Rief W, Barke A, Aziz Q, Bennett MI, Benoliel R, Cohen M, Evers S, Finnerup NB, First MB, Giamberardino MA, Kaasa S, Kosek E, Lavand'homme P, Nicholas M, Perrot S, Scholz J, Schug S, Smith BH, Svensson P, Vlaeyen JWS, Wang SJ. A classification of chronic pain for ICD-11. Pain. 2015 Jun;156(6):1003-1007. doi: 10.1097/j.pain.0000000000000160. PMID: 25844555; PMCID: PMC 4450869.
5. Clinical diagnostic criteria and norms, functional diagnosis and capacity assessment of work on the basis of which the placement is made in the I, II and III degrees of disability, Annex to GD 1.542/2022, Official Gazette no. 1243 bis/22.12.2022, pg 4-5
6. Annex to Government Decision no. 1.542/2022 for approving clinical diagnostic criteria and norms, functional diagnosis and capacity of work assessment on the basis of which the placement is made in degrees I, II and III of disability, MO Nr. 1243 bis, 2022, pg 242-246

CHAPTER 2

ANKYLOSING SPONDYLITIS

SIMONA LIANA SOARE AND IOANA SOARE

Ankylosing spondylitis is a rare disease, the main representative of Spondylarthritis, which also include SpA associated with psoriasis, SpA associated with inflammatory bowel diseases.

ASAS-Assessment of Spondylarthritis International Society established the term of SpA Spondylarthritis in 2009, instead of Seronegative Spondylarthritis. SpA were classified according the type of joint evolvement:

I. Axial predominant SpA
   1. nr-ax-SpA: non-radiographic axial SpA
   2. ankylosing spondylitis AS
II. Peripheric predominant SpA
   1. reactive arthritis
   2. SpA associated with psoriasis
   3. SpA associated with Crohn disease or ulcerative colitis
   4. Juvenile SpA [1]

AS is a chronic inflammatory condition, affecting the axial skeleton with starting point at the level of the sacroiliac joints - bilateral sacroiliitis first and subsequently the spine in an ascending manner.

Over time, some patients may have peripheral joint damage: hips, knees, ankles (30%) [2]

Frequently it is associated with extraarticular manifestations: ocular, cardiac, pulmonary.

AS affect predominant young males between 20 to 40 years.

The characteristic anatomopathological element is enthesitis (inflammation of the insertion site of the ligaments and tendons on the bone), which leads to the destruction of the vertebral angles with subsequent ossification of the edges of the vertebral discs and immobilization of the spine).

AS is the most frequently associated with a genetic marker, the histocompatibility antigen HLA B27 in a proportion of 90-95%, but only 50% of individuals presenting HLA B27 develop AS. The most important risk factor for AS is HLA B 27. The presence of HLA B 27 in the population is 8%.

Patients with HLA-B27 negative are diagnosticated with delay.

In the initial stage of the disease, inflammation is active, and early treatment could prevent the appearance of new inflammatory lesions and the development of syndesmophytes responsible for ankylosing the spine with repercussions on the functional capacity of the patient with AS.

Untreated, it can lead to the immobilization of the spine with severe dorsal kyphosis, with significant damage to the excursions of the ribcage during breathing, which in time leads to restrictive respiratory insufficiency. Can lead to immobilization in flexion of the cervical spine with severe limitation of the visualization of the environment.

AS is a disease of the young adult, who is usually male, of an active age. This fact justifies the attempt to prevent the occurrence of the joint immobility and the disability.

At the beginning, the vertebral pain caused by the inflammation is the main symptom, that appears at night, accompanied by sweating and makes rest impossible.

To recognize the condition more easily and start the appropriate treatment early, in order to prevent the occurrence of irreversible damage caused by inflammation, the ASAS criteria were developed.

The **ASAS** (Assessment of Spondylarthritis international Society) criteria identify axial spondylarthritis (SpA when a patient under 45 years, presents with lumbar pain for minimum 3 months) and is found in one of the two situations:

1. Has **documented sacroiliitis** and associates:

    a. Inflammatory spinal pain
    b. Peripheral synovitis objectified by the physician
    c. Calcaneal enthesitis
    d. Anterior uveitis diagnosed by the ophthalmologist
    e. Dactylitis
    f. Psoriasis
    g. Inflammatory bowel chronic disease (or ulcerative colitis)
    h. Good response to anti-inflammatory drugs
    i. Family history of AS
    j. HLA-B27 present
    k. Increased CRP

2. The presence of HLA-B27 positive and the existence of at least two of the manifestations listed above, even if there are no sacroiliitis changes on MRI or radiography.

If until now the presence of HLA B-27 was only considered a high susceptibility to the disease, currently the presence of this genetic marker is considered a diagnostic criterion.

The English rheumatologist of Romanian origin, Andrei Calin, showed many years ago the main characteristics of the inflammatory spinal pain (Bath criteria):

- The pain has an insidious onset
- Is persistent for at least 6 weeks
- It is accompanied by prolonged morning stiffness which can last up to 3 hours
- Is accentuated after prolonged rest
- Improves with physical exercise and NSAID administration

The functional evaluation can also be performed using the ASAS criteria, including BASDAI **(Bath Ankylosing Spondylitis Disease Activity Index) [1].**

Evaluation / Monitorization

Physical function	BASFI or Functional Index Dougados
Pain	VAS/NRS last week for spine, nocturne
Spine mobility	Excursions of the ribcage during breathing Shober test Anterior flexion, lateral flexion Occiput -wall distance
Global evaluation of patient	VAS/NRS last week
Matinal	Duration in the spine last week
Fatigue	VAS last week
Peripheral joints/enthesis	Nr. of swollen joints out of 44 joints Enthesitis index
Inflammation tests	CRP, ESR
Spine RG	Lumbar: ant/post and lateral Cervical: lateral Pelvis for sacroileal joints

*BASFI - Bath AS Functional Index; NRS - Numerical Rating Scale; VAS - Visual Analogue Scale; RG – radiography

In patients with axial involvement the pain intensity is measured with VAS or NRS

The assessment of functional involvement is done with BASFI.

The activity of the disease is assessed with BASDAI and ASDAS (Ankylosing Spondylitis Disease Activity Index).

BASDAI comprises 6 questions:

1. The level of the fatigue – VAS: 0-10; 0-absent; 10 -very severe
2. Description of the cervical, lumbar, hip pain: 0-10
3. Description of the pain and the other joints swelling: 0-10
4. Description of the pain determined by the pressure in different zones: 0-10
5. The severity of the morning stiffness
6. The duration of the morning stiffness

*For 5 and 6 we make the average

We divide the sum of questions 1 to 6 by 5:

A score >4 means an active disease

A score <2 a mild activity of the disease

ASDAS -Ankylosing Spondylitis Disease Activity Score is composed of 5 variables, lumbar pain, the duration of morning pain and stiffness, VAS: 0-10 which assess the pain in the last week, the swollen joints, and CRP (mg/L)

- ASDAS > 3,5 = disease with very high activity
- ASDAS >2,1 and <3,5 disease with high activity
- ASDAS >1,3 and < 2,1 disease with moderate activity
- ASDAD < 1,3 non active disease

Non-radiographic axial SpA – represents a subtype of SpA, without structural sacroiliac changes. In these patients MRI may reveal the inflammatory changes at the level of sacroiliac joints and in the enthesis, which are responsible for the pain and the reduced quality of life. It is possible that this non-radiographic entity represents a previous stage in the evolution of AS. Studies documented that 5-10% of non-radiographic axial SpA patients will develop radiographic sacroiliitis in the following 2 years and 20% will develop AS in 5 years.

The progression factors for the development to AS are: positive HLA-B27, elevated CRP, bone edema visualized on MRI, buttock pain, anterior uveitis and smoking.

Treatment

Considering the occurrence of this disease in young men, the treatment must be focused on returning to work and increasing the quality of life, as well as on slowing down the evolution and preventing the complications.

AS being a chronic condition with a high degree of disability, it requires the initiation of recovery therapy from the initial stage and continuous physical exercise, independent of the evolution of the disease.

The main objectives of the rehabilitation treatment in AS patients are:

- pain relief
- maintaining or improving joint mobility
- strengthening of the paravertebral muscles, pectoral muscles, hip adductors and hamstrings

- toning the abdominal muscles and the paravertebral muscles, the iliopsoas muscle, the gluteal muscles, the quadriceps muscles
- maintaining the pulmonary functional capacity
- improving the patient's quality of life
- encouraging the return to work.

Among all the physical-kinetic means (thermotherapy, laser, electrotherapy, hydrotherapy, massage, kineto-therapy), only kineto-therapy demonstrated a significant contribution to the achievement of these objectives.

The physiotherapy program can be carried out by the following methods:

1) Corrective postures and exercises and awareness of body alignment.

The tendency of the disease is to determine the anteflexion of the head, dorsal kyphosis, lumbar lordosis with anteversion of the pelvis and flexion of the hips, therefore the prevention or correction of these changes will be pursued.

2) Exercises to increase the flexibility of the cervico-dorsal-lumbar spine and the belts, assisted by the therapist, involving stretching techniques for synergistic muscles and suppling techniques for the periarticular tissues.
3) Active exercises with light resistance for toning the paravertebral, abdominal muscles, the gluteus and the iliopsoas - which by its action is a lordosant.
4) Respiratory reeducation. Affecting the dorsal vertebral segment and the costovertebral joints by the inflammatory process limits the expansion of the ribcage and determinates the installation of the syndrome of chronic restrictive respiratory insufficiency.

It is insisted on increasing inspiration through appropriate positioning, by coupling the movements of the upper limbs with those of the trunk. In this way, regional thoracic openings are made that facilitate inspiration. The diaphragm will be toned by the contraction and relaxation of the abdominal wall with counter pressure. In the ante- and retropulsion movements of the abdominal wall, an important role is played by the toning of the transverse abdominal muscle. Breathing training exercises, also focused on inspiration, will be performed daily.

5) Hydrokinetic therapy can be applied including in cases of exacerbation of the disease, the benefits of movement in hot water being well

known: pain relief, general mental and muscular relaxation, weight loss, increased joint mobility, etc.

Medication

At the beginning the only therapy was the administration of NSAIDs, respiratory gymnastics and mobilization of the spine. Now there are multiple ways and medications available for the physician.

1. NSAIDs lower the inflammation, relieves pain and improves spine mobility. We utilize diclofenac 150mg/day, naproxen 1000mg/day, indometacin75-100/mg/day; new NSAIDs specific inhibitors of COX2 (celecoxib, etericoxib), have a better digestive tolerance and can be administered for long periods.
2. Glucocorticoids are usually administered locally intraarticular in peripheral inflamed joints and in enthesis.
3. Sulfasalazine can be administered in AS with peripheric arthritis.
4. Biological:

In recent years biological therapy with TNFα inhibitors -adalimumab, infliximab, golimumab, certolizumab and inhibitors of TNFα receptors – etanercept, were introduced in order to halt the local inflammatory process (enthesitis) more quickly, and stop spinal lesions [5].

The indication of this therapy are for patients with severe inflammatory syndrome and in cases of rhizomelic damage [3].

A monoclonal antibody against IL17 was introduced in the therapy of AS-Secukinumab.

The response to therapy is monitored by using BASDAI and ASDAS.

A comparison of the score is done between the initial values obtained at the start of therapy and the scores after 3 months of treatment = delta ASDAS; if the score is >1,1 then there is an important clinical improvement, and if it is more than 2 then it represents a major clinical amelioration.

The initiation of biological therapy is done according to EULAR recommendations when the patient with AS has high values of CRP, inflammatory signs in the sacroiliac joint on MRI or Radiography and when the patient did not respond to conventional treatment with 2 NSAIDs drugs for 4 weeks, or sulphasalazine in peripheric form, and has a high activity of the disease: ASDAS >2,1 and BASDAI > 4.

In ocular involvement -anterior uveitis- anti TNFα drugs (Adalimumab) are useful for patients who did not respond well or not at all to corticosteroid therapy or have contraindication to corticosteroid treatment.

In the administration of this therapy, the possibility of an increase in the incidence of neoplasia, infections and the reactivation of tuberculosis must be considered [3].

In very severe forms of AS surgical treatments are recommended, such as: osteotomies and arthroplasties.

Rating

+75 to +100 for active SpA [2].

Standard rates may be accepted for inactive disease (minimum 1 year without therapy and without significant spinal deformity).

Patients with marked spinal deformity, ankylosis of the hips or shoulders, or those with aortic incompetence, heart conduction defects or with protein excretion in urine less than 2g/24h will require an additional rating of +50 to +150 [2]. Patients with protein excretion in urine more than 2g/24h should be declined [2].

Criteria for disability in Romania [12]

Slight functional deficiency 20-49%

I. Ankylosing spondylitis / non-radiographic central form -axial spondylarthritis in **sacroiliitis phase**
II. Ankylosing spondylitis /non-radiographic axial spondylarthritis central form with **gripping the sacroiliac joint and the dorso-lumbar spine.**
III. Ankylosing spondylitis / non-radiographic axial peripheral spondyloarthritis form at onset.

No activity limitation or mild limitation

No restrictions/slight restrictions on participation in social life.

It requires health services for curative treatment and slowing down the evolution of the disease, and a recovery program (physio-kinetics therapy).

Education and training services may be required, vocational and employment counseling.

Medium functional deficiency 50-69% - Invalidity 3rd degree

I. Ankylosing spondylitis / non-radiographic axial spondylarthritis central form with **gripping of cervico-dorso-lumbar spine**
II. Ankylosing spondylitis/non-radiographic axial spondylarthritis mixed form or peripheral with gripping of large peripheral joints - knees, elbows, with joint stiffness.

Moderate limitation of activities, especially during developmental stages.

Moderate restrictions on participation in social life, especially during exacerbations.

It requires health services for curative treatment, prevention of complications and slowing down the evolution of the disease, recovery program (physio-kinetics therapy) - care and rehabilitation services in the long term.

Social assistance services are needed. Some general social support services may also be required.

Accentuated functional deficiency 70-89%- Invalidity 2nd degree

I. Ankylosing spondylitis / non-radiographic axial spondylarthritis central form with clamping of the cervico-dorso-lumbar spine and **fixation of the cervical spine in flexion.**
II. Ankylosing spondylitis / non-radiographic axial spondylarthritis central form with **fastening of scapulo-humeral or coxo-femoral belts**.
III. Ankylosing spondylitis / non-radiographic axial spondylarthritis **peripheral form** with gripping of large peripheral joints - knees, elbows, fists with severe disorders of locomotion or gesture.

Moderate / severe limitation of activities.

Severe restrictions on participation in social life.

It requires health services for curative treatment, prevention of complications and slowing down the evolution of the disease, recovery program (physio-kinetics therapy) - care and rehabilitation services in the long term.

Social assistance services are needed. Some general social support services may also be required.

Severe functional deficiency 90-100% - Invalidity 1st degree

I. Ankylosing spondylitis / non-radiographic axial spondylarthritis central form with clamping of the cervical spine and the scapulo-humeral and coxo-femoral belts bilaterally with tendencies to ankylosis in vicious positions.
II. Ankylosing spondylitis / non-radiographic axial spondylarthritis mixed forms or severe peripheral with multiple ankylosis (**knee in flexion; tibiotarsus ankylosis in equine, etc.).**

Severe/complete limitation of activities.

Complete restrictions on participation in social life.

Requires health services for treatment, possibly providing devices (devices for self-service, crutches, frames, wheelchairs, etc.), assistive technologies and other adapted equipment (arrangement of the home and access ways).

Services of social assistance are required. Some general social support services and also accompanying persons or personal assistants may be necessary [12].

References

1. Rudwaleit M, van der Heijde D Landewe R Akkok N, Brandt J, Chou CT et al. The Assessement of Spondyloarthritis Classification International Society classification criteria for peripheral sponddyloarthritis and for spondyloartyritis in general. Ann Rheum Dis 2011 Jan,70(1):25-31
2. Brackenridge RDC, Elder W John, Medical Selection of Life Risks, 4th Edition, Macmillan reference Ltd, 1998, p 834-835
3. Fallahi S, Jamshidi AR Diagnostic Delay in Ankylosing Spondylitis; Related factors and prognostic outcomes
4. Maxwell LJ, Zochling J, Boonen A, Singh JA, Veras MMS, Tanjong Ghogomu E, Benkhalti Jandu M, Tugwell P, Wells GA - Anti-TNF-alpha drugs for treating ankylosing spondylitis; https://www.cochrane.org/CD005468/MUSKEL_anti-tnf-alpha-drugs-for-treating-ankylosing-spondylitis
5. Braun J, Sieper J. Ankylosing spondylitis. Lancet 2007; 369(9570): 1379-1390.

6. Dougados M, Baeton D. Spondylarthritis. Lancet 2011; 377(9783): 2127-2137.
7. Braun A, Saracbasi E, Grifka J, Schnitker J, Braun J. Identifying patients with axial spondyloarthritis in primary care: how useful are items indicative of inflammatory back pain? Ann Rheum Dis 2011;70(10):1782-1787.
8. Rudwaleit M, Jurik AG, Hermann KG et al. Defining active sacroiliitis on magnetic resonance imaging (MRI) for classification of axial spondyloarthritis: a consensual approach by the ASAS/OMERACT MRI group. Ann Rheum Dis, 2009;68(10):1520-1527.
9. Sieper J, Rudwaleit M, Baraliakos X et al. The assessment of Spondylo Arthritis International Society (ASAS) handbook: a guide to assess spondyloarthritis. Ann Rheum Dis, 2009;68 Suppl 2:ii1-ii44.
10. Rudwaleit M, Listing J, Brandt J, Braun J, Sieper J. Prediction of a major clinical response (BASDAI 50) to tumour necrosis factor alpha blockers in ankylosing spondylitis. Ann Rheum Dis 2004;63(6):665-670.
11. Tam LS, Gu J, Yu D. Pathogenesis of ankylosing spondylitis. Nat Rev Rheumatol 2010;6(7):399-405.
12. Annex to Government Decision no. 1.542/2022 for approving clinical diagnostic criteria and norms, functional diagnosis and capacity of work assessment on the basis of which the placement is made in degrees I, II and III of disability, MO Nr. 1243 bis, 2022, p 242-246

CHAPTER 3

PSORIATIC ARTHRITIS

SIMONA LIANA SOARE AND IOANA SOARE

PsA is heterogeneous in terms of skin and joint manifestations, the severity of these manifestations and the coexistence of various clinical forms.

There is a temporal relationship between the debut of articular and skin lesions, in most cases (approximately 75%) arthritis starts when psoriasis is already diagnosed and is clinically viewed as an evolutionary situation of the psoriatic disease. There are situations in which skin and joint involvement occur simultaneously - 10% of cases. The most difficult context for diagnosis is when arthritis precedes the skin lesion - 15% of cases, extending the time to a correct diagnosis [1].

The CASPAR (The Classification of Psoriatic Arthritis) study [1] which included 588 patients versus 536 controls took into account the subtypes of arthritis and defined inflammatory joint disease as the situation in which a minimum of 3 points of the following are accumulated:

Criteria	Score
Manifestations of Psoriasis	2
Personal history of psoriazis seen by the doctor	1
Family history of psoriasis	1
Dactilytis	1
New bone juxtaarticular formation	1
Negative RF	1
Nail dystrophy	1

Clinical Manifestations

I musculoskeletal

1. **Arthritis** - monoarthritis to polyarthritis

Moll and Wright classification contains 5 subgrups of PsA: DIP joint only, asymmetrical oligoarthritis, symmetrical polyarthritis, spondylitis, mutilans arthritis

A. DIP joint only- pathognomonic for PsA-evolution to erosive forms of arthritis;

Frequently associates dactylitis and nail psoriasis changes; local enthesitis is also present;

B. asymmetrical oligoarthritis- 11-70% at the beginning of the disease-implies small joints of the hands and feet - especially DIP and big joints like tibiotarsal joints;

C. symmetrical polyarthritis- >4 joints -small joints of hands and feet-60%;

D. spondylitis - axial involvement 20-40-%-the same main clinical manifestations as in AS: lower back pain for >3 months, during the night and early morning-inflammatory pain with morning stiffness for at least 30 minutes. The pain has a good response to NSAIDs and improves with exercise;

E. mutilans arthritis - the rarest but most severe form of psoriatic arthritis causes bone loss in the affected joints, which can make it impossible to bend or straighten them; the fingers become shortened by arthritis, and the shortening may become severe enough that the hand looks paw-like, with the first deformity occurring at the interphalangeal and metacarpian-phalangeal joints. The excess skin from the shortening of the phalanx bones becomes folded transversely as if retracted into one another like opera glasses, hence the description **la main en lorgnette.** As the condition worsens, dislocation, phalangeal and metacarpal bone absorption, and skeletal architecture loss in the fingers occur. Sometimes, in addition, there is foot involvement in which toes can shorten and develop painful calluses in a condition known as **opera glass foot, or pied en lorgnette**.

EULAR guidelines approach management of psoriatic arthritis from the perspective of the rheumatologist. They focus on pharmacological treatments for musculoskeletal manifestations and make recommendations for treatment targets and outcome measures. In cases of substantial skin involvement, EULAR recommends working closely with a dermatologist.

The GRAPPA recommendations provide a treatment plan that outlines the specific therapeutic pathways tailored to the domains involved: peripheral arthritis, axial disease, enthesitis, dactylitis, skin and nails.

2. **Enthesitis** - represents the **inflammation of tendons or ligament insertions on bone or the joint capsules on bones** and is followed by bone erosions and local bone proliferation.

The most affected are: the Achilles tendon, the site of insertion of plantar fascia on calcaneum and ligament insertions on the pelvis. Very useful in the detection or confirmation of enthesitis are musculoskeletal US and MRI. The presence of these clinical manifestations is associated with radiologic progression of axial and peripheral joints.

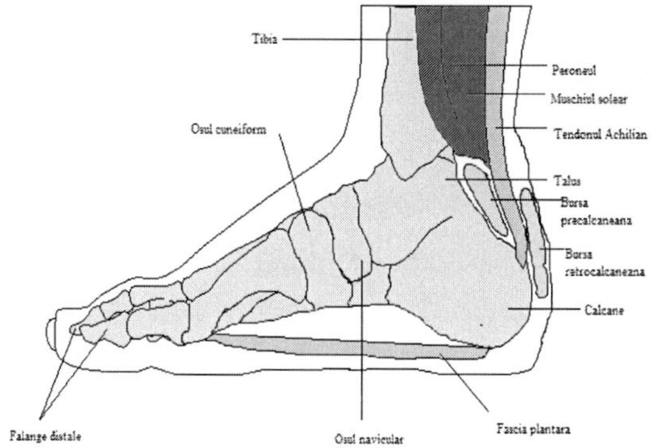

Fig. 1 Normal aspect [3]

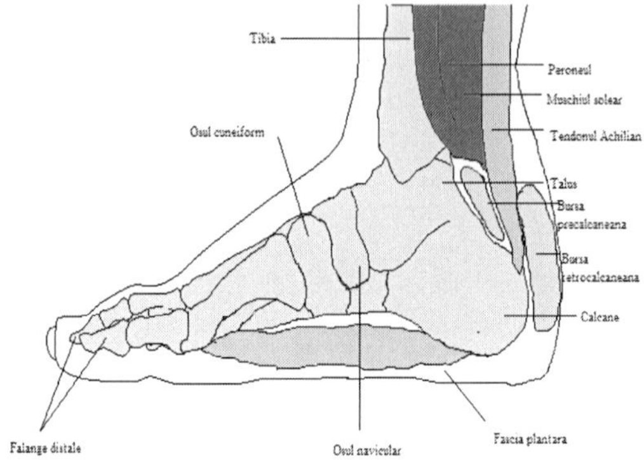

Fig. 2 Plantar Fasciitis, Achilles tendinitis and pre- and retrocalcaneal bursitis [3].

3. **Dactylitis-sausage fingers-** characteristic for PsA 30-50% of patients

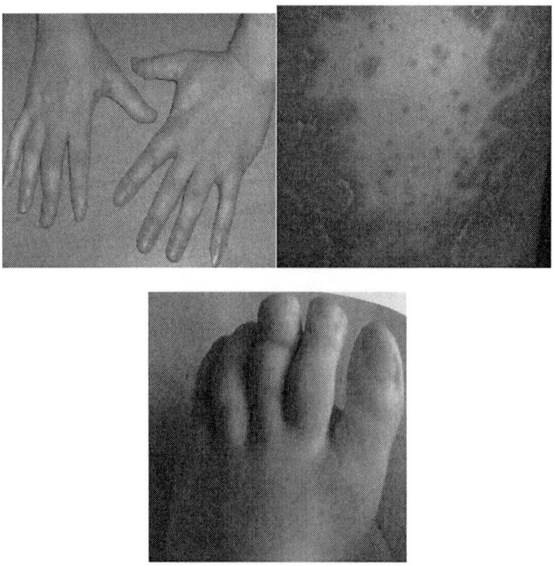

Fig. 3 Dactylitis (Archive of Prof. Călin Giurcăneanu, Dermatology, Elias Hospital)

Asymmetrically affecting several fingers. More frequently in the toes than in the fingers.

It is a factor of bad prognosis and is frequently associated with erosive forms of arthritis.

II Extra-skeletal manifestations 49% prevalence

1 Skin manifestations

Squamous-erythematous plaque-specific lesion-which has various dimensions, with detachable scales, which when removed, causes bleedings.

Most common sites: joint extension zones, elbows, knees, scalp, retroarticular, umbilical, nails and around the nails, buttocks.

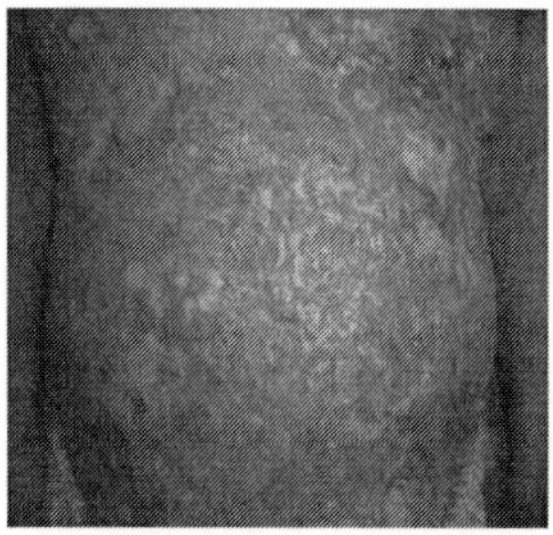

Fig.4 Vulgar psoriasis of the abdomen (on the left) and posterior thorax (on the right) (Archive of Prof. Călin Giurcăneanu, Dermatology, Elias Hospital)

2 Nail involvement - can be the only lesion - affecting 80% of PsA patients and 30%–50% of PsO patients, and consists of:

- **Onycholysis** is the gradual, painless separation of a nail from the underlying nail bed. The pocket created can form a pathway for bacteria or fungi to infect the nail bed. About one-third of people with nail psoriasis develop a fungal infection
- **Nail pitting** (these depressions on the nail are the most common symptom of PsA, occurring in more than two-thirds of people with the disease, according to the Psoriasis and Psoriatic Arthritis Alliance, they can be small and shallow or big and deep.)
- **Subungual** (underneath a finger or toenail) **hyperkeratosis**
- **Ridging-** Inflammation of the matrix (the area at the base of the nail where the cells that produce new nail growth are produced) can cause these grooves and ridges that run lengthwise and are known as Beau's lines. They usually occur on every fingernail or toenail.

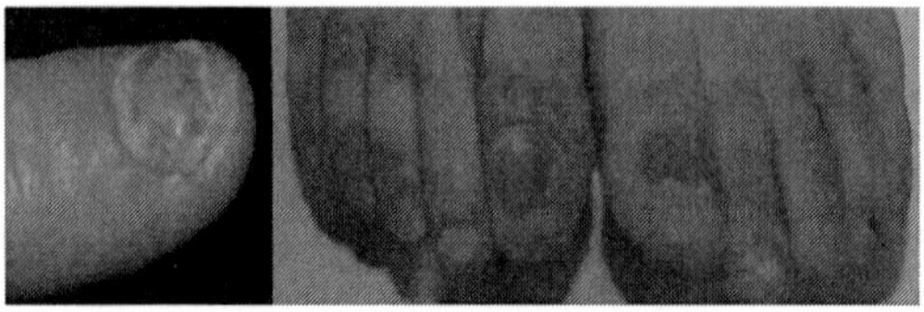

Fig. 5 Nail psoriasis (Archive of Prof. Călin Giurcăneanu, Dermatology, Elias Hospital)

3 Ocular involvement

- **Conjunctivitis** - present in 20%of patients - good prognosis
- **Uveitis** - present in 7% of patients; starts insidious, is bilateral and rather continuous
- **Episcleritis** - rarely
- **Sicca syndrome** - usually secondary

4 Intestinal involvement - asymptomatic and symptomatic when a patient may present an inflammatory disease type - Crohn's.

5 Cardiac involvement - rarely: aortitis, aortic regurgitation

6 Rare manifestations- IgA nephropathy, amyloidosis, pulmonary fibrosis, myopathy.

Laboratory

Inflammatory tests: increased ESR, CRP, and fibrinogen, especially in the polyarticular subgroup where a mild rise of RF- 2-10%, and anti-CCP antibodies 8-16% can be identified.

Radiologic examination can reveal: the arthritis in the phalanges with symmetrical distribution, the involvement of DIP, the absence of juxta-articular osteoporosis, the phalangeal marginal erosions and in mutilans arthritis the proximal phalangeal osteolysis- "pencil in cup".

In the axial forms, there are syndesmophytes (calcifications) or heterotopic ossifications inside the spinal ligaments or in the vertebral annulus fibrosus, which is unilateral asymmetric. The inflammatory sacroiliac involvement is unilateral.

Ultrasound can identify the hyperaemia as an indirect sign of inflammation and the joint changes, especially enthesitis in the Achilles tendon [5].

MRI is done for the symptomatic patients to identify early the changes in the bones and enthesis.

Differential diagnosis can also be made depending on the patient's age:

1. up to 20 years with:
   a. rheumatic fever
   b. juvenile arthritis,
   c. infectious arthritis,
   d. Legg-Calve-Perthes deforming osteochondritis.
2. 20-40 years with:
   a. vertebral discopathy,
   b. spondylolisthesis,
   c. inflammatory arthritis,
   d. septic arthritis,
3. over 40 years with:
   a. vertebral discopathy,
   b. spondylolisthesis,
   c. inflammatory arthritis,
   d. osteoporosis,
   e. metastases [3].

Evolution

- Undulating, with exacerbations and remissions.
- If the patient benefited from the therapies that prevent the joint deformation, the risk of mutilating arthritis would be reduced to 5%.

Discussion

In most patients, the psoriatic skin lesions precede arthritis or develop concomitantly with it. In 15% of cases, the rheumatological manifestations precede the skin involvement [4]. This subset of patients with psoriatic arthritis “sine psoriasis” can be identified by the presence of spondyloarthropathy with dactylitis and/or distal interphalangeal arthritis, HLA-Cw6 and a family history of psoriasis.

Careful examination of the patient and a systematic search for “hidden” psoriasis lesions are important for the diagnosis of erosive arthritis, often mutilating. The presence of rheumatoid factor does not exclude the diagnosis of psoriatic arthritis (it is positive in 5% of cases).

To assess the activity of the disease in the predominantly axial form, the BASDAI index (Bath Ankylosing Spondylitis Disease Activity Index) is used, which analyses the degree of fatigue; the degree of pain in the cervical, dorsal or lumbar spine; the degree of pain and swelling in the peripheral joints; how pain was felt when touching or pressing on the painful areas - the enthesis and the degree of morning stiffness. All these parameters are estimated on a scale from absence to very severe.

The natural evolution of psoriatic arthritis is progressive and worsens over 10-20 years. The exacerbations, during which the pains are exacerbated, decreasing the degree of mobility and increasing the tendency to ankylosis in some vicious positions, are followed by the periods of calm of 1-2 years. The functional deficit worsens after each surge, reducing the joint mobility and limiting the movement possibilities, affecting both their professional and their social life.

The severe evolution is associated with young age, female gender, and severe joint involvement.

Comorbidities: metabolic syndrome, carotid atheromatosis, obesity.

The functional capacity in the psoriatic arthritis can be lost to varying degrees depending on the clinical phenotype. Psoriatic arthritis, presenting as asymmetric oligoarthritis with involvement of small joints—such as IFD in the hands or feet—and mild skin involvement, typically results in mild functional deficiency. This is associated with a mild adaptive disability of 20-49% while still preserving the patient's working capacity, following the criteria from Romania [9].

Psoriatic arthritis in the form of asymmetric oligoarthritis with the involvement of a single large joint or 2-3 small joints associated with the psoriasis skin lesions, leads to average functional deficiency with the adaptive incapacity of 50-69% and a loss of at least half of the work capacity, falling into the III degree of disability.

Psoriatic arthropathy in the form of psoriatic spondylitis, with axial involvement of the cervico-dorso-lumbar spine, associated with ankylosis and hand deformation (claw hand) is responsible for the accentuated functional deficiency with the adaptive incapacity of 70-89% and with the total loss of work capacity, giving II degrees of disability.

In the terminal phase, the bone ankylosis is reached, and the muscle stiffness, the fibrocapsular retraction and the bone proliferation (joint blockage) determine a drastic reduction in the patient's quality of life, with a reduction in self-service capacity and dependence, the patient falling into the first degree of disability [9].

Rating varies from 0 to 150+ [10].

Prognostic

Factors for an unfavorable prognosis:

- onset at a young age
- acute onset
- extensive skin involvement (Popa L, 2012)
- polyarticular involvement
- presence of the HLA DR4, HLA DR3, HLA B27 pattern
- associated HBV, HCV, HIV infection

The mortality is not significantly increased (Gladmann DD, 1995).

The functional prognosis: the disease can progress to fibrous or bony ankylosis of one or more joints (Magalhães RF, 2010).

Treatment

Aims - to smooth the evolution, to prevent the handicap.

The drugs used are NSAIDs, local glucocorticoids and csDMARDS, bDMARDS [11,12,13,14].

1 NSAIDs - inhibitor drugs of cyclooxygenase 1: Indomethacin, Diclofenac, Ketoprofen, Piroxicam.

NSAID inhibitor drugs of cyclooxygenase 2: Celecoxib, Etoricoxib.

NSAIDs are used to control the pain and the inflammation.

2 Corticoids - are administered in severe forms of disease to control the inflammation and the pain till the DMARDS begin to start their effect.

3 csDMARDs - Methotrexate 15-25mg/week -in the polyarticular subtype, Leflunomide

1. Sulfasalazine - SSZ 2-3g/day when the patients have no response to treatment using MTX or Leflunomide

2. Apremilast - phosphodiesterase inhibitor - more efficient than csDMARDS and bDMARDs. It is administered when there is not a good response to csDMARDS and the patients have contraindications to bDMARDS.

3. bDMARDs - biologic disease-modifying anti-rheumatic drugs

   This biological therapy has changed the outcome of these patients by stopping the progression of destructive arthritis and alleviating the symptoms.

   The indications for this kind of therapy are the severe cases of the disease: the erosive polyarticular subtype, the lack of remission with standard therapy or a mild activity of the disease under classic DMARDs

   In the axial subtype, the biologics are administered, if there is a lack of response to NSAIDs.

   The biologics approved for PsA are the inhibitors of IL17A-secukinumab or the inhibitors of IL12/23-ustekinumab.

   TNFα inhibitors- the monoclonal antibody IgG1-Infliximab, which is administered with MTX. A good response to treatment is represented by a decrease in skin lesions and joint involvement. In addition, the PASI (Psoriasis Aria and Severity Index) and DAPSA - the score of disease activity, will also decrease.

   Adalimumab - human monoclonal antibody anti-TNFα has the same response.

   Certolizumab - improves joint and skin lesions.

   Etanercept - exogenous soluble receptor for TNFα improves only arthritis.

   Golimumab - human monoclonal antibody anti-TNFα greatly improves enthesitis, nails and skin lesions and the quality of life.

   Secukinumab - human monoclonal antibody type IgG1/k which neutralises pro-inflammatory IL17A.

Monoclonal antibodies: Ixekizumab = anti Il17A and Ustekinumab-anti Il 12 - involved in the inflammatory response of Th1and Il23 involved in Th17 activation.

4. Inhibitors of JAK-kinase - an alternative to the biologic drugs; oral Tofacitinib inhibits cytokines by affecting JAK 1 and 3.

Contraindicated to patients with a previous history of venous thrombosis and pulmonary embolism.

Only for skin involvement (all other medications act on both skin and joint lesions), we use retinoids and photo-chemotherapy PUVA.

EULAR recommendations [14]

1. Non-steroidal anti-inflammatory drugs should be used in the monotherapy only for mild PsA, and in the short term, the oral glucocorticoids are not recommended.
2. In patients with peripheral arthritis, the rapid initiation of conventional synthetic disease-modifying antirheumatic drugs is recommended and Methotrexate is preferred.
3. If the treatment target is not achieved with this strategy, a biological disease-modifying antirheumatic drug (bDMARD) should be initiated without preference among modes of action. Relevant skin psoriasis should orient towards bDMARDs targeting the interleukin (IL)-23p40, IL-23p19, IL-17A and IL-17A/F inhibitors.
4. In the case of predominant axial or entheseal disease, an algorithm is also proposed. The use of Janus kinase inhibitors is proposed primarily after bDMARD failure, taking the relevant risk factors into account, or in case bDMARDs are not an appropriate choice.
5. Inflammatory bowel disease and uveitis, if present, should influence the drug choices, with the monoclonal tumor necrosis factor inhibitors proposed.
6. Drug switches and tapering in sustained remission are also addressed.
7. These updated recommendations integrate all currently available drugs in a practical and progressive approach, which will be helpful in the pharmacological management of PsA.

Conclusions

Following the epidemiological studies conducted in Europe and North America, we consider psoriasis to be a disease with a high frequency in the population, 2-3%, with psoriatic arthritis occurring in 30% of these cases. Modern management of this chronic systemic inflammatory disease must target not only skin involvement but also joint involvement.

Patients with psoriasis should be carefully consulted and investigated with imaging (entheseal ultrasound, MRI) to detect joint damage in order to achieve early diagnosis and early, adequate, more aggressive treatment in the presence of psoriatic arthritis, which therefore will prevent the occurrence of disability.

It has been found that psoriatic arthritis has comorbidities, and we must identify the patients at risk for metabolic disorders and cardiovascular diseases to correct the risk factors and treat the associated conditions.

The quality of life of these patients can significantly be improved by the psychological interventions.

References

1. Taylor W, Gladman D, Helliwell P, Marchesoni A, Mease P, Mielants H; CASPAR Study Group Classification criteria for psoriatic arthritis: development of new criteria from a large international study. Arthritis Rheum. 2006 Aug; 54(8):2665-73.
2. Acosta Felquer ML, FitzGerald O Peripheral joint involvement in psoriatic arthritis patients Clin Exp Rheumatol. 2015;33(5 Suppl 93):S26-30.
3. Soare SL, Psoriatic Arthropathy, Etna Publishing House, 2013, 978-973-1795-51-5
4. Alamanos Y, Voulgari PV, Drosos AA Incidence and prevalence of psoriatic arthritis: a systematic review. J Rheumatol. 2008;35(7):1354.
5. Moll JM, Haslockl, Macrae IF, et al.Associations between ankylosing spondylitis, psoriatic arthritis, Reiter's disease, the intestinal arthropathies, and Behcet's syndrome. Medicine (Baltimore) 1974;53:343-64.
6. Peluso R, lervolino S, Vitiello M, Bruner V, Lupoli G, Di Minno MN. Extra-articular manifestations in psoriatic arthritis patients. Clin Rheumatol. 2015 Apr;34(4):745-53.
7. Fojtikova M, Stolfa J, Novota P, Cejkova P, Dostal C, Cerna M. HLA-Cw*06 class I region rather than MICA is associated with psoriatic arthritis in Czech population. Rheumatol Int. 2009;29(11):1293-9.
8. Acosta Felquer ML, Santiago Ruta S, Rosa J et al. Ultrasound entheseal abnormalities at the distal interphalangeal joints and clinical nail

involvement in patients with psoriasis and psoriatic arthritis, supporting the nail-enthesitis theory. Semin Arthritis Rheum. 2017 Dec;47(3):338-342.

9. Clinical diagnostic criteria and norms, functional diagnosis and capacity assessment of work on the basis of which the placement is made in the I, II and III degrees of disability, Annex to GD 1.542/2022, Official Gazette no. 1243 bis/22.12.2022, pg 4-5
10. Brackenridge RDC, Elder W John, Medical Selection of Life Risks, 4th Edition, Macmillan reference Ltd, 1998, p 835
11. Fitzgerald O, Winchester R. Psoriatic arthritis: from pathogenesis to therapy. Arthritis Res Ther. 2009;11(1):214.
12. Mease PJ. Biologic Therapy for Psoriatic Arthritis. Rheum Dis Clin North Am. 2015 Nov;41(4):723-38.
13. Smolen JS, and all. Treating axial spondyloarthritis and peripheral spondyloarthritis, especially psoriatic arthritis, to target: 2017 update of recommendations by an international task force. Ann Rheum Dis. 2018 Jan;77(1):3-17.
14. Gossec L, Baraliakos X, Kerschbaumer A, et al. EULAR recommendations for the management of psoriatic arthritis with pharmacological therapies: 2019 update. Ann Rheum Dis. 2020; 79:700-712.

CHAPTER 4

BRAIN TUMORS - EVALUATION AND TREATMENT PROBLEMS

IOANA SOARE AND ROXANA MIRICA

Introduction

Cancer is a large group of diseases that can start in almost any organ or tissue of the body when abnormal cells grow uncontrollably, go beyond their usual boundaries to invade adjoining parts of the body and/or spread to other organs [1]. For the last 100 years, cancer was defined only based on histogenesis - cells of origin or similar microscopic features. In the classification of brain tumors, immunohistochemical characteristics were later added, and after 2016, also molecular parameters [2].

In time, there were multiple classifications of the brain tumors.

Brain tumors are divided into benign, more recently called "non-malignant" and malignant [1], primary and metastatic.

In the brain we can have metastasis, sometimes as the only sign of presence of cancer in the organism.

World Health Organization (WHO) Description of brain tumor grades [3]:

Grade I: These are the least malignant tumors and are usually associated with long-term survival. They grow slowly and look almost normal when viewed under a microscope.

Grade II: These tumors grow slowly and appear slightly abnormal under a microscope. Some may spread to nearby normal tissue.

Grade III: These tumors are malignant, although there is not always a significant difference between grade II and grade III tumors. The cells of a grade III tumor are actively reproducing, they are abnormal cells, which grow in the nearby normal brain tissue.

Grade IV: The most malignant tumors reproduce rapidly, invading nearby normal brain tissue. These tumors form new blood vessels so that they can maintain their rapid growth. They may have an area of necrosis in the center [3,4].

Brain tumors are considered rare diseases, taken each type separately, although there are over 120 different types of primary brain tumors [1,9].

Nearly one-third (29.7%) of brain and central nervous system (CNS) tumors are malignant [1, 4,5].

In the USA, between 2013 and 2017, in people over the age of 40, brain tumors were the 8th most common cancer and the third cause of cancer death [5].

As with any rare disease, according to EURORDIS, the correct diagnosis can take between 5 and 30 years [6,7]. These patients do not have so much time. Brain tumors have as their first symptom a headache, a quite common polymorphic symptom. This does not help to quickly diagnose this type of condition [5,6,7].

Sometimes the patient suffers a minor craniocerebral trauma, performs a brain CT or MRI, on which occasion asymptomatic brain tumors are highlighted. Sometimes you discover the cancer only at the autopsy, as reveils a study from Japan, where up to 24% of sudden unexpected cancer deaths have a definite diagnosis only post-mortem [8].

This poses particular problems in cases of brain neoplasms, because early detection and early treatment increase the life expectancy of these patients.

Therefore, many brain and CNS neoplasms are diagnosed in late stages, clinically and imaging, and the biopsy is no longer performed.

Obtaining treatment based on health insurance - problems in practice

Any patient with normal tissue biopsy, although on imaging may have multiple space-occupying formations, with a clear malignant appearance, invasive, cannot be classified as a cancer patient and does not benefit from specific treatment. Some oncologists resolve the uncertainty based on clinical and imagistic criteria, in support of the patient's access to treatment.

Any patient with a biopsy, diagnosed with borderline tumor, grade 2-3 (borderline 2), cannot receive cancer treatment because he does not meet the criteria for malignancy.

All patients in whom biopsy is not possible (deep layer tumor, high risk of bleeding, multiple tumors, life expectancy below 3 months [11]) have virtually no definite cancer diagnosis and cannot receive specific treatment.

These patients cannot receive oncological treatment or radiotherapy because of the restrictive indications of the insurers (health insurance companies) or because of the risk of allegations of malpractice. Patients will not receive some social security rights (short term sick leave, disability pension) in the same way as cancer patients, but only as a patient with a common illness [12]. Patients can receive palliative treatment, can be hospitalized in oncology departments.

Presentation of clinical cases

Case 1: A 57-year-old male doctor fainted in hospital following surgery for a hernia and suffered a minor brain trauma (2019). A brain MRI was performed urgently, which did not detect hematomas or other acute lesions, but highlighted: lesion in the right hippocampus, 3 / 2cm, which makes common body with the choroid plexus of the right lateral ventricle and develops in the right parietal white matter, formation in the left lateral ventricle 1cm, lesion in the anterior horn of the right lateral ventricle of 0.8cm, multiple lesions "in oil stain" with contrast substance lining the ventricles (including proximal 1/3 of the brainstem), a meningeal lesion in the upper portion of the cerebellar vernix.

After 2 weeks, he underwent a neurosurgical intervention for diagnostic purposes, with a superficial tumor biopsy, a biopsy limited by a bleeding of multiple neovessels. The biopsy indicated normal brain tissue.

The blood tests were normal, with no signs of inflammation (ESR 2mm/h, fibrinogen 317 mg / dl), only with 19% eosinophilia. The patient had no other diseases. The differential diagnosis was made with CNS tuberculosis [13,14], parasitosis, because the MRI result was extremely polymorphic. The patient was asymptomatic for another 2 months after the biopsy, then complained of altered general condition, memory disorders, slowness in speech, loss of appetite. After 3 months from the diagnosis, another MRI and a cerebral angio-MRI were performed, observing the tumor growth by about 30% on each lesion. The opinions of the imaging doctors consulted, ranged from a choroid plexus papilloma or a malignant tumor, including a glioblastoma.

Because of the defensive medicine, no biopsy result, polymorphic lesions, the patient was refused by several oncologists and received only palliative treatment.

Motor disorders with unsafe gait appeared 10 months after diagnosis, requiring hospitalization. The patient died in a palliative care ward 11 months after the revealing accident.

The patient could not obtain medical leave for 548 days with 100% payment, as for oncological diseases, but only 183 days with 80% of the salary, as for a common illness (in Romania). He obtained a disability pension 6 months after the onset of the disease, based upon neurological signs and imaging, the diagnosis being "Multiple brain tumors".

Case 2: A 27-year-old male patient, operated for a borderline astrocytoma (glioblastoma), classified as a grade 2 tumor after the biopsy, presented to the insurance medicine office for Long-Term Sick Leave- disability pension. This patient also did not benefit from medical leave for oncological disease and was retired based on neurological signs. The diagnostic for invalidity pension was „Borderline brain tumor, operated". The patient's evolution was undulating, with recurrences. The patient obtained oncological treatment after insistence, because there is no practical difference between grade 2 and grade 3 tumors, as states Aldape, Mansouri and colleagues in an article published in 2015 and the WHO Description of brain tumor grades [3,4,15,16].

Case 3: A 45-year-old male patient with a tumor located near the base of the skull, in an area inaccessible for biopsy, inoperable, invasive, discovered late, presented for disability pension. It was considered to have virtually no diagnosis. He did not receive oncological treatment. He was retired based on neurological syndromes, the diagnosis being "Inoperable brain tumor". The evolution was quickly unfavorable.

Discussions

The cancer model based solely upon histological findings is obsolete, especially for patients with brain tumors. The non-biopsiable patients can be diagnosed by other means, as cell-free circulating tumor DNA, used in non-small cell lung cancer and other malignant conditions [17].

Piccionni and all found ctDNA in 50% of meningiomas and glioblastomas, in a study in 419 patients, published in 2019 [18].

Non-biopsiable patients and their doctors may receive another help from AI, artificial intelligence.

Computer -assisted Physician Documentation/ computer-aided medical diagnostic (CAD) were developped as early as 1950. In 1998, the first commercial CAD system for mammography, the ImageChecker system, was approved by the US FDA. In the following years several commercial CAD systems for analyzing mammography, breast MRI, medical imagining of lungs, colon, and heart also received FDA approvals. Currently, CAD systems are used as a diagnostic aid to provide physicians for better medical decision-making [19,20].

A big progress was accomplished from 2015 till now in Computer Vision and Machine Learning, part of Artificial Intelligence. Imagenet project from 2009 gathered big data [21]. Because of the scientific collaboration in its realization, all this data is openly available for scientists. A lot of Neural Network applications were developed.

Convolutional Neural Network is one such application used for object recognition model. Steps for predictive modelling were huge. Now scientists use deep learning models in the cloud.

YOLO (You Only Look Once) system is an open-source method of object detection that can identify objects in images and video. In the last years the program got from 20s per image to 20 ms per image, so 1000 times faster, allowing very interesting medical applications, as real time image analyze in endoscopy, ophthalmology [22,23]. This computer assisted image analyze was better and more accurate than the human one, allowing small lesions detection [22].

Wang and Wu 2010 Results in Pathological brain detection (PBD), analyzed over 160 images. They showed that the classification accuracy was 98.75% [24].

In 2014, Padma et al. used combined wavelet statistical texture features to segment and classify AD benign and malignant tumor slices [25].

Such progress may help develop a new diagnosis protocol for such non-biopsiable cases of brain tumors. This might reduce the time interval from the symptoms appearance to the diagnostic, as biopsy is usually hard to obtain and time consuming.

Should we rely only on computer tumor recognition? Probably not. But computers will perform in the future a more accurate and thorough exam of the brain CT, SPECT, PET or MRI imaging as a human, due to longer exam time, small detail detection, complete exam, and not least, due to huge databases embedded.

Conclusions

Brain tumors are extremely polymorphic and therefore are considered rare diseases (each type affects less than 1 person in 2000). Brain tumors are a very common cause of cancer death in patients under the age of 40 (in the USA), and therefore must be more actively diagnosed.

Patients with brain tumors may have the following issues: tumors are in deep or vital regions; they refuse the biopsy; the neurosurgeon does not reach the tumoral tissue and the biopsy is irrelevant; advanced cases, considered "outside the surgical and oncological therapeutic resources". These patients cannot receive oncological treatment or radiotherapy because of the restrictive indications of the insurers (health insurance companies) or because of the risk of allegations of malpractice. The lack of a biopsy should not prevent the patient in obtaining cancer treatment, nor in obtaining social security rights.

Patients will not receive some social security rights (short term sick leave, disability pension) in the same way as cancer patients, but only as a patient with a common illness. Patients can receive palliative treatment, can be hospitalized in oncology departments.

I propose to neurologists and oncologists to develop a diagnostic and treatment protocol, based on imaging aspects for these non-biopsiable cases, which will still offer a chance at specific oncological treatment, with increased life expectancy. Computer Vision, Neural Networks and Deep Learning Models may offer in 2 years time diagnostic tools to differentiate non-malignant from malignant tumors of the central nervous system, for the non -biopsy cases. We can use also some laboratory criteria - (ctDNA).

It is not normal that in the 21st century we cannot overcome these barriers. It is not normal to leave patients untreated, and we are not just referring to neurosurgical treatment, which may not be indicated sometimes.

Disclaimer: This Chapter was first published in a reduced form as an article in Austin Journal of Clinical Neurology, Volume 8 Issue 2-2021.

References

1. https://www.who.int/en/news-room/fact-sheets/detail/cancer, access 02.04.2021
2. David N. Louis, Arie Perry and all, The 2016 World Health Organization Classification of Tumors of the Central Nervous System: a summary https://braintumor.org/wp-content/assets/WHO-Central-Nervous-System-Tumor-Classification.pdf access 20.04.2021
3. https://www.abta.org/about-brain-tumors/brain-tumor-education/#:~:text=Brain%20Tumor%20Statistics&text=Over%20700%2C000%20Americans%20are%20living,primary%20brain%20and%20CNS%20tumors access 30.03.2021
4. https://www.hopkinsmedicine.org/neurology_neurosurgery/centers_clinics/brain_tumor/diagnosis/brain-tumor-grade.html access 30.03.2021
5. Ostrom QT, Patil N, Cioffi G, Waite K, Kruchko C, Barnholtz-Sloan JS. CBTRUS Statistical Report: Primary Brain and Other Central Nervous System Tumors Diagnosed in the United States in 2013–2017. Neuro Oncol. 2020.
6. https://www.cancer.org/cancer/brain-spinal-cord-tumors-adults/detection-diagnosis-staging/detection.html access 30.03.2021
7. https://www.eurordis.org/ access 30.03.2021
8. Hideto Suzuki, Takanobu Tanifuji, Nobuyuki Abe, Tatsushige Fukunaga, Characteristics of Sudden Unexpected Cancer Deaths Investigated by Medical Examiners in Tokyo, Japan 2009, Published online 2014 Mar 5. Prepublished online 2014 Jan 25. J Epidemiol. 2014; 24(2): 141–145. doi: 10.2188/jea.JE20130087, PMCID: PMC3956693, PMID: 24463959, https://www.ncbi.nlm.nih.gov/pmc/articles/PMC3956693/,

access 05.04.2021
9. http://www.cnas.ro/page/programul-national-de-tratament-pentru-boli-rare.html access 30.03.2021
10. http://www.orpha.net/national/RO-RO/index/despre-boli-rare/ access 30.03.2021
11. https://neurocentrum.ro/cum-se-trateaza-metastazele-cerebrale/ access 30.03.2021
12. Ioana Soare, Medical Expertise. Insurance Medicine, Etna Publishing House, 2017, ISBN 978-973-1985-08-4, Bucharest, Romania
13. Adriana Hristea, Tuberculoza sistemului nervos central, 2018, ISBN 9786065241992, CTEA Publishing House, Romania
14. Petru-Emil Muntean, Tubercular meningitis, http://pneumon.org/assets/files/789/file771_664.pdf, acces 27.04.2021
15. Teodora Camelia Vladescu, Modern Criteria in the Glial Tumors Classification, 2005, Etna Publishing House, Bucharest, Romania, ISBN 973-87046-9-3, 20-31, 70-72.
16. Aldape K, Zadeh G, Mansouri S, Reifenberger G, von Deimling A. Glioblastoma: pathology, molecular mechanisms and markers. Acta Neuropathol. 2015 Jun;129(6):829-48. doi: 10.1007/s00401-015-1432-1. Epub 2015 May 6. PMID: 25943888. https://pubmed.ncbi.nlm.nih.gov/25943888/
17. Marina Kushnir, Carmen Murias,and all, Journal of Clinical Oncology 2018 36:15_suppl, e24044-e24044
18. Piccioni DE, Achrol AS, Kiedrowski LA, et al. Analysis of cell-free circulating tumor DNA in 419 patients with glioblastoma and other primary brain tumors. CNS Oncol. 2019;8(2):CNS34. doi:10.2217/cns-2018-0015
19. Doi K. Computer-aided diagnosis in medical imaging: historical review, current status and future potential. Comput Med Imaging Graph. 2007;31(4-5):198-211. doi:10.1016/j.compmedimag.2007.02.002
20. https://en.wikipedia.org/wiki/Computer-aided_diagnosis access 23.04.2021
21. www.image.net.org acces 25.04.2021
22. Junfeng Gao, 1,2,3 Yong Yang, 4 Pan Lin,1,2,3 and Dong Sun Park, Computer Vision in Healthcare Applications, Journal of Healthcare Engineering 2018:1-4 DOI: 10.1155/2018/5157020
23. YOLOv2: https://arxiv.org/pdf/1612.08242v1.pdf
24. https://towardsdatascience.com/yolo-you-only-look-once-real-time-object-detection-explained-492dc9230006, access 23.04.2021

25. Padma, A.; Sukanesh, R. (2014). "Segmentation and Classification of Brain CT Images Using Combined Wavelet Statistical Texture Features". Arabian Journal for Science and Engineering. **39** (2): 767–776. doi:10.1007/s13369-013-0649-3. S2CID 62615810.

CHAPTER 5

INVALIDITY EVALUATION IN COVID-19

CONSTANTIN GHIMUȘ,
PARASCHIVA POSTOLACHE,
ROXANA MIRICA AND IOANA SOARE

The first reports of the prolonged symptoms after COVID-19 emerged in the spring of 2020, when patients and the medical community noticed that some individuals continued to experience health problems (more than 3 months), long after their tests for the virus had turned negative. In June 2020, the World Health Organization (WHO) officially recognized Long COVID as a distinct condition, paving the way for further research and the development of clinical guidelines for diagnosis and treatment. It is named also: Post-COVID Conditions, long-haul COVID, post-acute COVID-19, long-term effects of COVID, chronic COVID, post-acute sequelae of SARS CoV-2 infection (PASC).

Epidemiology

Epidemiological studies indicate that between 10% and 30% of people infected with the SARS-CoV-2 virus develop persistent symptoms lasting more than four weeks after the initial infection [1]. Although these numbers may vary depending on the population studied and reporting methods, it is clear that long COVID represents a substantial burden on health systems and patients.

Not all people infected with SARS-CoV-2 develop long-term COVID, and the predisposition to this condition seems to be influenced by several factors. Studies suggest that women are more likely than men to experience long-term symptoms of COVID [2]. Also, people with preexisting comorbidities such as obesity, diabetes, and cardiovascular disease are at greater risk of developing the condition [3]. Older age is also a risk factor, although long COVID can also affect young and healthy people.

Risk factors

Risk factors for developing long COVID include initial severity of COVID-19 disease, with patients who required hospitalization or intensive care having a higher risk (4). However, long COVID can also occur in individuals with mild forms of the initial infection. A high viral load and /or a dysfunctional immune response may contribute to the risk of having long COVID [5].

Etiopathogeny

The precise mechanisms by which long COVID develops are not fully understood, but research suggests that multiple pathophysiological pathways may be involved. One theory is that SARS-CoV-2 infection can lead to persistent systemic inflammation and an abnormal immune response that can affect multiple organs and systems [6]. It has also been suggested that long COVID could involve direct damage caused by the virus at the cellular level, as well as side effects of treatments used in the acute phase of the disease. Other possible mechanisms include microvascular dysfunction, autoimmunity, and reactivation of latent viruses.

Clinical manifestations

The most commonly reported symptoms include:

1. Fatigue: It is one of the most common and debilitating symptoms, often described as extreme fatigue that does not improve with rest [2].
2. Dyspnea: breathing difficulties persist in many patients, even with normal radiologic aspect in the lungs [4].
3. Chest pains: Are common and may be attributed to the persistent inflammation or to the damage to the heart muscle.
4. Cognitive problems (brain fog): many patients report difficulty concentrating, memory loss and other cognitive deficits [7].
5. Myalgias and arthralgias: muscle and joint pains are common and can significantly affect the quality of life [8].
6. Digestive disorders: diarrhea, nausea and abdominal pain may persist in some patients [5].
7. Psychological symptoms: Frequently reported are anxiety, depression and sleep disturbances [6].

Paraclinical evaluations

The diagnosis of long COVID is mainly clinical, based on history and the presence of persistent symptoms after acute infection. However, various paraclinical evaluations are often necessary to rule out other causes and to assess the multisystemic impact of the condition. Among the most common paraclinical investigations are:

1. Lab tests: Blood tests can reveal persistent inflammation, through markers such as CRP and ESR. Liver and kidney function tests are also important, to rule out other pathologies [1].
2. Chest radiography and computed tomography (CT): are used to evaluate any structural abnormalities in the lungs and to rule out any persistent pulmonary complications [4].
3. Pulmonary function tests: spirometry and respiratory function testing are essential to assess respiratory capacity and detect possible lung dysfunction [9].
4. Magnetic Resonance Imaging (MRI): Brain and cardiac MRI can be used to investigate neurological and cardiovascular symptoms, providing detailed information about inflammation or tissue damage [7].
5. Echocardiography: This is useful for assessing cardiac function and detecting any structural or functional abnormalities of the heart [10].
6. Neuropsychological tests: these are used to assess cognitive function and to document cognitive deficits reported by patients [11].

Diagnosis

The diagnosis of long COVID is mainly based on the history and the identification of persistent symptoms that appear at least four weeks after the initial infection with SARS-CoV-2.

1. Detailed history: involves the timing and severity of the initial SARS-CoV-2 infection. It is also important to document any comorbidities and previous treatments [6].
2. Symptom assessment: main symptoms such as fatigue, dyspnea, chest pain, cognitive impairment and other systemic symptoms will be identified and quantified [1].
3. Laboratory tests: although there are no specific markers for long COVID, blood tests can be useful to assess systemic inflammation (CRP, ESR) and organ function (liver and kidney tests) [4].

4. Functional and imaging tests: Investigations such as spirometry, lung diffusion tests, chest x-ray, computed tomography (CT) and magnetic resonance imaging (MRI) can be used to assess functional and structural damage to various organs [10].

Differential diagnosis

A comprehensive assessment is crucial to avoid misdiagnosis and ensure appropriate treatment.

1. Chronic Fatigue Syndrome (CFS/ME): Symptoms of extreme fatigue and cognitive dysfunction are common in both CFS/ME and long COVID. The differential diagnosis is based on the history of recent infection with SARS-CoV-2 and the exclusion of other causes [2].
2. Lung conditions: Dyspnea and fatigue can be found in chronic lung diseases, such as asthma, chronic obstructive pulmonary disease (COPD) and pulmonary fibrosis. Functional and imaging tests are essential to differentiate these conditions [9].
3. Cardiovascular disease: Chest pain and shortness of breath can be symptoms of cardiovascular disease, such as heart failure and coronary heart disease. Echocardiography and electrocardiogram (ECG) are important to exclude these pathologies [10].
4. Neurological and psychological disorders: Cognitive disorders and psychological symptoms can be found in neurological and psychiatric conditions such as depression, anxiety and encephalopathy. Neuropsychological evaluations and psychiatric consultation can help clarify the diagnosis [7].
5. Autoimmune and inflammatory conditions: Systemic symptoms and joint pain can occur in autoimmune diseases. Autoimmune tests (ANA antibodies, rheumatoid factor) can be useful in ruling out these conditions [6].

Prognosis

Long-term COVID prognosis varies considerably among individuals, depending on the initial severity of SARS-CoV-2 infection, the presence of comorbidities, and the specificity of persistent symptoms. In general, studies show that long COVID symptoms can persist for months and, in some cases, even more than a year. However, most patients experience gradual improvement over time.

1. Duration of symptoms: Studies indicate that between 20% and 30% of patients with long COVID continue to have significant symptoms six months after initial infection (4).
2. Severity of symptoms: symptoms can range from mild to severe, and patients with more severe forms of COVID-19 appear to be at greater risk of developing long COVID [6].
3. Recovery: Although many patients report an improvement in symptoms over time, some may be left with permanent sequelae, especially if they have had severe complications such as lung or heart damage [10].

Treatment

Long COVID treatment is largely symptomatic and individualized, focused on relieving symptoms and improving patients' quality of life. Therapeutic approaches include:

1. Respiratory rehabilitation: Respiratory recovery programs are essential for patients with dyspnea and other persistent respiratory problems. These include breathing exercises and adapted physical activity [9].
2. Fatigue management: Behavioral interventions, such as cognitive behavioral therapy (CBT), and energy conservation techniques can help manage severe fatigue [2].
3. Psychological support: Counseling and therapy can be beneficial for patients experiencing anxiety, depression and other psychological symptoms. Social support and support groups are also important [6].
4. Pharmacological treatments: Anti-inflammatory drugs and pain relievers can be used to control symptoms such as muscle and joint pain. In severe cases, more specific interventions such as corticosteroids for persistent inflammation may be required [5].
5. Cognitive rehabilitation: cognitive rehabilitation programs are used to help patients with memory and concentration problems by providing techniques and exercises to improve cognitive function [7].

Prevention

Prevention of long COVID is based on prevention of initial infection with SARS-CoV-2 and appropriate management of acute infection. Strategies include:

1. Vaccination against COVID-19 is the most effective way to prevent infection and, by implication, long COVID. [12].
2. Protective measures [13].
3. Early treatment can reduce the risk of long-term complications. The use of antiviral treatments and other evidence-based therapies may be crucial [6].

Impact on work capacity

Persistent symptoms, such as severe fatigue, brain fog, dyspnea, muscle aches and joint pain, can reduce the work performance and the ability to maintain a regular work schedule.

1. Extreme may affect up to 70% of patients [1], with a significant reduction in productivity, the need for frequent breaks or a reduced work schedule.
2. Cognitive disorders such as concentration difficulties and memory lapses can prevent patients from performing tasks that require attention to detail and complex cognitive skills [7].
3. Psychological symptoms: Anxiety, depression and other psychological disorders can also interfere with the ability to work effectively and contribute to frequent medical absences [6].

Long COVID and Insurance Medicine

Long COVID is a major challenge for health insurance systems and insurance medicine due to the variability of symptoms and prolonged recovery time. Managing this condition in the insurance context involves complex evaluations.

1. Assessment of work capacity: Insurance physicians must conduct detailed assessments to determine the long-term impact of COVID on patients' work capacity. These evaluations include a complete history, clinical examination, and additional testing to document the severity and persistence of symptoms [6].
2. Medical Documentation: Collecting and presenting adequate medical documentation, including specialist reports, laboratory and imaging test results, and psychological and functional assessments, is essential [3].
3. Extended sick leave: In many cases, patients with long COVID require extended sick leave. Health insurance and physicians must

work together to ensure continuity of financial support throughout recovery [14].

4. Work incapacity benefits: For patients whose ability to work is severely impaired in the long term, work incapacity benefits may be necessary. These are based on periodic assessments and continuous medical evidence of work incapacity [4].

Disability criteria

Early retirement due to long COVID involves meeting specific criteria, which vary from one jurisdiction to another, but are based on common principles.

1. Duration and severity of symptoms: Patients must demonstrate that their symptoms persist for an extended period, usually at least six months, and that these symptoms are severe enough to prevent continued work under normal conditions [15].
2. Multidisciplinary Assessment: Assessments for early retirement often require a multidisciplinary approach, including family physicians, infectious disease specialists, pulmonologists, neurologists and psychologists. This is necessary to provide a complete picture of the long-term impact of COVID on health status [10].
3. Functional disability: Assessment of functional disability includes tests of physical and cognitive performance. These may include walking tests, spirometry, standardized cognitive assessments, and other functional tests to document reduced work capacity [2].
4. Lack of improvement: To be eligible for early retirement, patients must demonstrate that their symptoms do not improve significantly despite adequate medical treatment. This is assessed by continuous monitoring and documentation of symptoms and treatment attempts [6].
5. Psychological and social impact: Assessments must also consider the psychological and social impact of long COVID on the patient's life. Psychological disorders such as anxiety and depression should be documented and considered in the context of overall work capacity [5].

How it happens in Canada:

Long-Term Disability (LTD) Benefits

If long COVID prevents you from working for an extended period, you may qualify for LTD benefits, which provide ongoing financial support until you're able to return to work or reach retirement age. Insurers require medical proof that your condition meets their definition of "total disability."

- Application: Requires detailed medical evidence and may involve assessments by the insurer.

Canada Pension Plan (CPP) Disability Benefits

If Long COVID symptoms are severe and prolonged, and prevent you from working, you may qualify for qualify for CPP disability.

- Application: Submit a detailed application and medical report to Service Canada.

Disability Tax Credit (DTC)

The DTC can help reduce the taxes you owe if long COVID severely impacts your daily life. It requires certification from a medical practitioner and approval from the Canada Revenue Agency.

- Application: Requires Form T2201 to be completed by you and your medical practitioner and submitted to the Canada Revenue Agency.

Provincial Disability Benefits

Every province in Canada has its own disability support programs, usually based on financial need and how severe your disability is. These programs may provide income support, health coverage, and employment services. However, proving Long COVID as a disability can be difficult, as the condition is new and often hard to diagnose.

- Application: Process varies by province, typically involving an application form and medical assessment [18].

Limitations

We do not have criteria to assess objectively fatigue, the most common symptom in PASC - there are only some subjective tests, such as Fatigue Severity Scale FSS, designed to differentiate fatigue from clinical depression, since both share some of the same symptoms. Essentially, the FSS consists of a short questionnaire that requires the subject to rate his or her own level of fatigue. The obvious problem with this measure is its subjectivity as it is a self-report scale [16].

We have no criteria for functional pain syndromes.

Covid-19 has no associated retirement criteria, at least in Romania.

Conclusions

Invalidity pension (long-term sick leave) is still rare in COVID-19. The information about it is scarce and fragmented.

The predictors for invalidity for patients with long COVID are sex (male), age over 50 years, prior sick leave, and inpatient care - all being non-medical factors.

In this review of the studies regarding patients with post-acute sequelae of SARS-CoV-2 infection (PASC), evaluated at 3 and 6 months mostly, assessment for disability was performed for lung damage (fibrosis), heart damage (cardiomyopathy), neurological sequels, and other disabling remnant affections (anxiety, depression).

Invalidity evaluation must be realised in total, not only from a psychiatric or respiratory point of view, for example, because Long COVID can be a multi-systemic disease.

We can evaluate globally the patient with the 6MWT, or perform some cardiopulmonary tests, but these investigations are not complete and do not reflect the disability or just the work capacity. The use of ICF is non-specific.

The studies used only subjective evaluation for fatigue (as Fatigue Severity Scale FSS) or pain (Visual Analogue Scale -VAS), high frequency persistent symptoms found before dyspnoea. We found no criteria to assess objectively fatigue - some proposed exercise tests, but the resulting information was limited.

The studies used for this review did not clearly define “severe” or “critical” Covid.

Patients with PASC/ Long Covid are still rare (13% in the Swedish cohort) and we cannot yet appreciate how many of them will need invalidity pension [17].

References

1. Sudre, C. H., Murray, B., Varsavsky, T., et al. (2021). Attributes and predictors of long COVID. Nature Medicine, 27, 626-631
2. Davis, H. E., Assaf, G. S., McCorkell, L., et al. (2021). Characterizing long COVID in an international cohort: 7 months of symptoms and their impact. EClinicalMedicine, 38, 101019.
3. Greenhalgh, T., Knight, M., A’Court, C., Buxton, M., Husain, L. (2020). Management of post-acute COVID-19 in primary care. BMJ, 370, m3026.
4. Carfi, A., Bernabei, R., Landi, F. (2020). Persistent Symptoms in Patients After Acute COVID-19. JAMA, 324(6), 603-605.
5. Peluso, M. J., Kelly, J. D., Lu, S., et al. (2021). SARS-CoV-2 and Mucosal Immune Responses in Post-Acute Sequelae of COVID-19. Infection and Immunity, 89(9), e00302-21.
6. Nalbandian, A., Sehgal, K., Gupta, A., et al. (2021). Post-acute COVID-19 syndrome. Nature Medicine, 27, 601-615.
7. Gorno-Tempini, M. L., Hillis, A. E., Weintraub, S., et al. (2021). Long COVID and the brain. Nature Reviews Neuroscience, 22, 534-535.
8. Nassari, S., Blaes, F., Pleyer, U., et al. (2021). Myalgia and arthralgia: Clinical characteristics of long COVID. Journal of Infection,
9. Mo, X., Jian, W., Su, Z., et al. (2021). Abnormal pulmonary function in COVID-19 patients at time of hospital discharge. European Respiratory Journal, 55(6), 2001217.
10. Mandal, S., Barnett, J., Brill, S. E., et al. (2021). Long-COVID: Understanding the recovery of patients with acute lung disease caused by SARS-CoV-2. Lancet Respiratory Medicine, 9(9), 1012-1024.
11. Alkodaymi, M. S., Omrani, O. A., Fawzy, N. A., et al. (2021). Prevalence of post-acute COVID-19 syndrome symptoms at different follow-up periods: A systematic review and meta-analysis. Clinical Microbiology and Infection, 27(5), 775-786.
12. Bergwerk, M., Gonen, T., Lustig, Y., et al. (2021). Covid-19 Breakthrough Infections in Vaccinated Health Care Workers. New England Journal of Medicine, 385, 1474-1484.

13. World Health Organization. (2021). COVID-19 advice for the public: Getting vaccinated. https://www.who.int.
14. Del Rio, C., Collins, L. F., Malani, P. (2021). Long-term Health Consequences of COVID-19. JAMA, 324(6), 603-605.
15. Kemp, H. I., Corner, E., Colvin, L. A. (2021). Chronic pain after COVID-19: implications for rehabilitation. British Journal of Anaesthesia, 127(3), 315-317.
16. Fatigue Severity Scale FSS https://hwcdn.libsyn.com/p/4/d/d/4dde8090545dc1c9/Fatigue-Severity-Scale.pdf?c_id=36881411&cs_id=36881411&preview=1620057104&no-libsyn-stats=true&expiration=1620060704&hwt=3fef02f3d807a242ed7e769ab36bca76
17. Westerlind, E., Palstam, A., Sunnerhagen, K.S. et al. Patterns and predictors of sick leave after Covid-19 and long Covid in a national Swedish cohort. BMC Public Health **21,** 1023 (2021). https://doi.org/10.1186/s12889-021-11013-2
18. https://stlawyers.ca/law-essentials/long-covid-disability-benefits-canada/

CHAPTER 6

PATIENTS IN INTENSIVE CARE UNITS: ACCESS TO DISABILITY PENSION

SALIM CAMER

1. Introduction

A serious illness is one of the most challenging trials a person can face. For patients in intensive care units (ICUs), the road to recovery is often long, arduous, and uncertain, with potential long-term effects on physical and mental health. In many cases, recovery is incomplete, leaving significant impairments that prevent these patients from returning to work due to the severity of their conditions [1]. Understanding eligibility for disability pensions becomes essential to provide financial and emotional stability during this difficult time, enabling these individuals to continue chronic treatment and live with dignity despite major disabilities [2].

2. The impact of ICU stays on patients with severe conditions

ICU patients often face extremely severe medical conditions. Many require intubation, mechanical ventilation, parenteral feeding, central venous access, and prolonged immobility, causing:

- **Prolonged physical disabilities**: Bedsores, chronic pain, respiratory conditions, muscle atrophy, orthopedic sequelae, paralysis, and plegias [1].
- **Cognitive impairments**: ICU delirium or Post-Intensive Care Syndrome (PICS) can cause memory loss, concentration difficulties, chronic fatigue, and psychological stress [1,4].
- **Mental health issues**: Depression, anxiety, and post-traumatic stress disorder (PTSD) are common among ICU survivors [4].

> "Patients with severe illnesses admitted to ICUs, regardless of the cause, often experience generalized deconditioning with renal, digestive, musculoskeletal, neurological, endocrine, cardiovascular, dermatological, psychological, and respiratory consequences. Among these, muscle strength loss is observed in over 50% of cases, peaking in the first 2–3 weeks" [1,4,5,6].

These effects significantly impact a person's ability to work, making external support mechanisms—such as disability or sickness pensions—crucial for financial, medical, and emotional support.

3. Eligibility for disability pensions

Eligibility criteria for obtaining disability pensions vary by country but generally include:

I. **Medical evaluation**
Proof of a medically certified disability affecting work capacity, documented by specialists and rehabilitation reports [3].

II. **Duration of disability**
A minimum duration (e.g., six months to one year) is usually required for disability benefits/pension [3]. Patients in ICU cannot wait for 6 months to obtain insurance and benefits.

III. **Work capacity assessment**
Patients may need evaluations to determine if they can perform any type of work, even with accommodations [3].

4. Disability grades in Romania

Under Romanian law, disability is classified into three grades:

- **Grade I**: Total loss of work capacity and autonomy, requiring caregiver assistance, if possible, with reduced professional activity [2,3].
- **Grade II**: Total loss of work capacity but retention of personal autonomy, with reduced professional activity.
- **Grade III**: Partial loss of work capacity, with reduced professional activity.

5. Steps for medical evaluation

1. Initial consultation

Referral to specialists for assessment of medical illness [3]. The vast majority of homeless individuals are brought to the Emergency Department (ED) by ambulance or SMURD, often following reports from passersby who find them collapsed on the street. Before labelling the situation as purely social, a complete clinical and paraclinical examination of the patient is absolutely mandatory. It is essential to determine whether the patient presents with an immediate life-threatening emergency (e.g., status epilepticus, severe alcohol withdrawal symptoms, delirium tremens, severe hypothermia, traumatic brain injuries, intoxications, etc.). If such conditions are identified, emergency medical intervention is required, and the patient can be transported to the hospital and admitted, even against their will, if they lack discernment and are in danger.

If the patient shows signs of impaired discernment (e.g., due to withdrawal symptoms or cognitive disorders), a psychiatric evaluation or multidisciplinary team assessment can be requested. According to Romanian legislation (Law no. 487/2002 on mental health), a person who poses a danger to themselves or others, and who lacks discernment, can be admitted without his/hers consent following legal procedures that uphold the patient's rights.

These situations require collaboration between multiple institutions and professionals, including: Medical personnel (emergency physicians, psychiatrists, neurologists), Psychologists, Social workers, Law enforcement/local authorities (if the individual exhibits aggressive behavior or poses a public threat, including assistance with transport), NGOs and addiction treatment centres. Subsequently, social services such as the General Directorate of Social Assistance and Child Protection (DGASPC) or non-governmental organizations can provide long-term support solutions, including housing, food, hygiene facilities, social reintegration, and treatment.

2. Compiling the medical file for retirement

Includes hospital discharge papers, test results and GP referrals.

3. Submission

Submit the documentation to the County Pension Office or the Bucharest Pension Office.

4. Evaluation by the medical committee

Includes clinical examination and review of documentation.

5. Issuance of disability decision

Disability may be permanent or temporary, with periodic re-evaluation [3].

6. Challenges in accessing disability pensions

- **Complex documentation**: Assembling all necessary documents is burdensome [5].
- **Lack of awareness**: Patients and physicians may not know about disability pension options [4].
- **Delayed recognition**: Cognitive or psychological impairments may emerge late.

7. Solutions for vulnerable populations

1. **Voluntary insurance**: Retroactive contributions for eligibility [4].
2. **Social assistance**: Guaranteed minimum income for those unable to contribute.
3. **NGO and local authority support**: Guidance and material aid [1].
4. **Disability allowance**: Certificates issued by DGASPC.
5. **Medico-Social Centers**: For continuous care [2].
6. **Social Housing**: Accommodations for vulnerable patients [2].

Integrated collaboration among hospitals, DGASPC, local institutions, and NGOs is vital to ensure social and legal protection for ICU survivors, in Romania.

DGASPC is the General Directorate of Social Assistance and Child Protection. It is a public institution in Romania, subordinated to county or local councils, responsible for

Social assistance: Providing services and support to vulnerable people, such as people with disabilities, the elderly, the homeless and families in difficulty.

The DGASPC works with other institutions and organizations to implement social assistance and child protection programmes, providing material, legal, psychological and medical support to those in need.

Globally, social centres such as Shelter and The Passage in the UK, Centre Médico-Social in France, and Mission Australia provide integrated services, including healthcare, housing, and rehabilitation. These models demonstrate the effectiveness of a multidisciplinary approach in addressing the complex needs of vulnerable populations. Adapting such frameworks in Romania could significantly improve outcomes for uninsured and homeless patients (International Labour Organization, 2021) [7,8.9.10,11,12].

In the last year, analysing the data obtained from the integrated system "Hipocrate" – discharges from the Clinical County Emergency Hospital of Constanta, we found out that a total of 1445 uninsured patients under the age of 65 were identified. As distributed by age and gender groups, the largest category is the age group 31-45 years with 202 females (40.66%) and 295 males (59.34%), followed by the age group 46-60 years, which includes 138 females (31.16%) and 305 males (68.84%). In the age group 19-30 years, 117 females (65.73%) and 61 males (34.27%) were recorded, while the age group 61-65 years includes 27 females (28.72%) and 67 males (71.28%).

The most common pathologies identified include mixed personality disorders (F61), with 80 cases (5.54%), acute pancreatitis (K85), with 32 cases (2.21%), and alcohol use disorders (F10.1), with 31 cases (2.15%). Other significant diagnoses include paranoid schizophrenia (F20.0), with 18 cases (1.25%).

In terms of the discharge destinations, patients were treated predominantly in General Surgery, for severe conditions such as sepsis and acute abdomen; Internal Medicine, for metabolic problems such as acidosis; Obstetrics-Gynecology for pregnancy-related complications; and Gastroenterology, for liver diseases such as alcoholic cirrhosis.

This distribution reflects the diversity of pathologies and medical needs, emphasizing the importance of a multidisciplinary approach for the effective care of patients in this category.

During the winter holidays, December 25-31, 2024, the Emergency Department, ED, of the Constanta Clinical County Emergency Hospital, faced considerable challenges in addressing the needs of uninsured or homeless patients. A total of 22 uninsured patients were registered, including six female patients and 12 male patients. Among these, one patient presented on four separate occasions during this period. Furthermore, five patients lacked any form of health insurance, while four patients had insurance specifically for chronic illnesses, allowing them to benefit from inclusion in the National Health Program for Chronic Diseases. Other patients are those receiving a disability or invalidity pension. In this category we only registered one patient.

Between December 25th and 31st, 2024, several measures were taken to address the needs of patients presenting to the Emergency Room. Two patients were admitted to Mangalia Hospital following the determined efforts of the emergency physician. Another two, diagnosed with osteoarticular tuberculosis, were transferred to the Agigea Osteoarticular TB Sanatorium. Additionally, two patients were admitted to Constanța County Emergency Hospital for further care and treatment. These cases underscore the critical role of collaboration between emergency services and specialized healthcare facilities in managing complex and urgent patient needs.

The **National Program for Chronic Diseases** addresses various medical conditions through specialized subprograms, including cardiovascular diseases, oncology, diabetes, neurological and endocrine disorders, rare diseases, mental health, and orthopaedics. It also covers treatment for hearing loss, liver failure, renal function supplementation for chronic kidney disease, haemophilia, thalassemia, and endometriosis, along with advanced diagnostic tools like PET-CT. This program ensures comprehensive care and support for patients with chronic conditions.

However, many patients admitted to the ED do not meet the criteria required for social services to file an application for their insurance, with the majority suffering from chronic alcohol abuse. These patients often lack the necessary documentation or a stable social situation, making it challenging to provide long-term solutions for their healthcare needs. Addressing this gap requires a coordinated effort between emergency services, social workers, and healthcare programs to ensure these vulnerable individuals receive the care and support they need.

Referring to the patients hospitalized in the ICU (intensive care unit) in the same period, we can say that out of the 46 cases, 16 cases were on Christmas days (December 25 and 26 with 6 patients per day, December 27 with 6 patients, December 27 with 4 patients, December 28 with 5 patients, December 29 and 30 with 7 patients/day, December 31 with 11 patients). 20 of them with maximum age of 65 years. Most of the patients were insured except for 4 uninsured patients and one insured patient with disability pension (oncologic patient). In all 4 cases, the patients are aged between 37-64 years old.

Another situation involves 10 uninsured or homeless patients currently hospitalized at the Constanța County Emergency Hospital. Of these, 3 patients have been hospitalized since April 2024, while 7 have been there since May 2024. Unfortunately, there are no local facilities available for their transfer or continued care. The only option at the national level is the **Medico-Social Assistance Unit in Bihor**, emphasizing the urgent need for additional resources and solutions to support such vulnerable individuals.

In Constanța, there is a social day shelter, **Sfânta Filofteia**, which can provide meals and hygiene services for patients. However, it does not have the capacity to offer medical care, highlighting the need for additional support systems to address both the medical and social needs of these vulnerable individuals.

In practical terms, regarding intensive care, patients admitted to that unit remain under the care of the department where they were initially hospitalized. Once their condition stabilizes and they no longer require intensive care, if they do not pass away, they are transferred to the corresponding department. At this stage, the coordinating physician, along with the head nurse and the social worker, works to find solutions for these patients.

Unfortunately, most patients remain on the hospital wards, resulting in significant costs for the hospital without providing a real solution for their situation. Many of these patients are uninsured, lack a stable home, or do not have family support to care for them. The transfer to a medico-social center, which could take over their care, is almost impossible because there is only one such center in the entire country, located in Bihor, as mentioned previously. This situation highlights the severe lack of infrastructure and resources needed to address the long-term care needs of vulnerable and unsupported patients effectively.

Conclusions

I truly believe that achieving these objectives does not require overly ambitious plans, but rather a collective commitment to building a more nurturing society. It is imperative that we do everything in our power to address these issues and acknowledge the unique importance of healthcare providers and the essence of humanity. Collective insight is both critical and pivotal for shaping the future of our healthcare system.

It is not a matter of debate that only insured patients have rights; rather, it is a fundamental truth that every human being has the right to health. By embracing this principle, we can move towards a more equitable and compassionate healthcare framework, ensuring that no one is left behind, regardless of their social or economic status.

References

1. Herridge, M. S., & Cameron, J. I. (2013). Disability after critical illness. New England Journal of Medicine, 369(14), 1367-1369.
2. World Health Organization. (2021). Report No. 534: ICU Survivorship and Disability.
3. Soare Ioana, Medical Expertise, Insurance Medicine, Handbook for the General Medicine Faculty, 2017, Etna Publishing House, p 72-75
4. Marra, A., Pandharipande, P. P., & Girard, T. D. (2017). ICU delirium and cognitive impairment: A tale of two syndromes. American Journal of Respiratory and Critical Care Medicine, 195(2), 134-141.
5. Needham, D. M., Davidson, J., Cohen, H., Hopkins, R. O., Weinert, C., Wunsch, H., ... & Harvey, M. A. (2012). Improving long-term outcomes after discharge from intensive care unit: report from a stakeholders' conference. Critical Care Medicine, 40(2), 502-509.
6. Elliott, D., Davidson, J. E., Harvey, M. A., Bemis-Dougherty, A., Hopkins, R. O., Iwashyna, T. J., & Needham, D. M. (2014). Exploring the scope of post–intensive care syndrome therapy and care: engagement of non–critical care providers and survivors in a second stakeholders meeting. Critical Care Medicine, 42(12), 2518-2526.
7. International Labour Organization (ILO). Social Protection Floors Recommendation No. 202. International Labour Organization, 2021.
8. European Observatory on Health Systems and Policies. Health Systems in Transition: Romania. European Observatory on Health Systems and Policies, 2021.
9. United Kingdom – The Passage. Integrating Healthcare and Housing Support for Vulnerable Populations: A Best Practice Model. The Passage, 2022.
10. Mission Australia. Mission Australia's Health and Housing Integration Programs. Mission Australia, 2023.
11. Centre Médico-Social (CMS). Post-Hospital Care and Social Reintegration in France: A Comprehensive Approach. CMS, 2022.
12. Romanian Government. Emergency Medical Assistance Law for Vulnerable Populations. Government of Romania, 2023.

CHAPTER 7

HEART FAILURE ASSESSMENT

PAUN NICOLAE AND IOANA SOARE

Heart failure does not have a clear definition. In the specialized literature, we find the congestive heart failure, the diastolic heart failure [1], the systolic or mixed heart failure, with the ejection fraction preserved (FE>50%), low (FE<40%) or slightly low (FE=41%-49 %), and last but not least, the cardio-respiratory insufficiency.

It can be acute, ephemeral (recurring or episodic) or chronic [2].

The European Society of Cardiology ESC adopted the following definition in 2021 [3]:

Heart failure is a clinical syndrome, in which patients have the following clinical signs:

1. Typical symptoms of heart failure
   - Shortness of breath
   - Fatigue and weakness
   - Edema of the ankles
2. Typical signs of heart failure
   - tachycardia,
   - tachypnea,
   - pulmonary rales
   - pleurisy,
   - increased pressure in the jugular veins,
   - peripheral edema,
   - hepatomegaly
3. Objective evidence of structural or functional changes of the heart at rest
   - cardiomegaly,
   - third heart sound,
   - heart murmur,

- abnormalities on echocardiography,
- increased concentration of natriuretic peptide.

Basically, heart failure is a syndrome triggered by a decrease in cardiac output that leads to hydro-saline retention in tissues or organs, followed by a decrease in tissue or organ perfusion [3].

Heart failure syndrome expresses the inability of the heart to ensure an adequate circulatory regime and represents the final stage in the evolution of all heart diseases. Cardiac damage occurs both as a result of diseases affecting the intrinsic cardiac structures (valves, coronary, myocardium, pericardium), but also through the action of extracardiac factors. We can mention here the heart failure from anemia, diabetes, chronic kidney disease, endocrine diseases, infiltrative or peripartum diseases, and others.

In anemias, the main mechanism that leads to heart failure is the decrease in the oxygen intake at the level of the myocytes, with the imbalance between intake and needs, all the more accentuated in patients with ischemic coronary disease. In these patients, the symptomatology is complicated.

Fatigue and even dyspnea are induced by both anemia and heart failure. Once the anemia is corrected, the symptomatology disappears completely, if there are no other heart diseases. If the clinical picture persists, even in a milder form, a pre-existing heart disease must also be considered. We would like to mention here the iron-deficiency anemia, which can generate symptoms, not only through the decrease of hemoglobin, but also through the very low levels of iron in the body. This can generate a discrepancy between the hemoglobin value and the degree of heart failure [3]. It should also be mentioned that, in general, only chronic anemia ends up being associated with heart failure. On another train of thought although some patients do not complain of fatigue or even shortness of breath, this is due to the fact that they involuntarily reduce the intensity of their daily effort. That's why an exercise test (even just walking fast or climbing the stairs) will reveal cardiac dysfunction. Fortunately, in the case of heart failure caused or aggravated by anemia, the clinical picture is completely reversible with the correction of the anemia and the removal of its cause, the patient regaining his previous functional capacity.

In the chronic kidney disease, the cardiac (cardio-vascular) damage that leads to increased mortality is mainly achieved by accelerating the atheromatous process and by valvular calcification, especially aortic stenosis. The lower the glomerular filtration rate, the more severe the cardiovascular damage and the higher the mortality [4]. That is why early detection and treatment of the kidney diseases is of the utmost importance, knowing that they are irreversible and have a progressive evolution.

In the same context, we can also include diabetes mellitus (DM), another major risk factor for cardiovascular diseases with the appearance of heart failure in the end. In addition to vascular damage, DM, especially uncontrolled type 2, often also associates with glomerulosclerosis. Thus, the mechanisms through which DM affects the vessels and the heart are multiple: dyslipidemia with the acceleration of atheromatous disease, micro- and macroangiopathy, arterial hypertension and last but not least, chronic kidney disease. Diabetic cardiomyopathy, although for a long time defined only echocardiographically by means of the Doppler examination, was demonstrated as a clinical entity with the help of the cardiac MRI examination [5]. It showed specific changes in the myocardium such as the increase in interstitial tissue mass as well as fibrosis and changes in capillaries and arterioles characterized by fibrous thickened walls. Thus, diabetic cardiopathy characterized by mild-moderate concentric hypertrophy with a non-dilated heart but with significant diastolic dysfunction is currently described. In the end, heart failure develops, often in the form of preserved EF, which quickly becomes disabling due to dyspnea and fatigue.

Regarding infiltrative diseases, the most common is amyloidosis. In this case, it is the infiltration of the myocardium, but also of other organs, with amyloid. This is a denatured protein of various origins, which loses its secondary and tertiary structure. Once deposited in the tissues, it cannot be metabolized and accumulates with irreversible damage to the function of the respective organ. In the case of the heart, there is an important ventricular hypertrophy with a marked decrease in diastolic function and cardiac output [6]. The most common forms today are amyloidosis from multiple myeloma or light chain disease in which fragments of lambda light chains are deposited in the form of amyloid. By treating the hematological condition, it can be stopped from evolving with a better prognosis. The second common situation is amyloidosis with transthyretin, the protein secreted by the liver that carries TSH. There can be a family form and a so-called wild (isolated) form. The evolution of heart failure is fast and the degree of disability of the patients is very high with very high mortality. Unfortunately, there are currently no effective treatments for cardiac amyloidosis.

In hyperthyroidism, heart failure most often occurs as a result of arrhythmias, and especially atrial fibrillation with a very fast heart rate [7].

Undetected in time, cardiac damage can develop with ventricular dilation and FE decrease, so-called reversible tachyarrhythmic cardiomyopathy, if it is detected in time. It should be mentioned that young patients tend to develop a clinical picture of hyperthyroidism without heart failure. In the elderly, who also associate other diseases, especially cardiac ones, the clinical picture of hyperthyroidism is blurred and incomplete, instead the phenomena of heart failure appear. The functional incapacity of the patients is important, due to the presence of the two conditions, hyperthyroidism and cardiopathy. Treated in time, hyperthyroidism is reversible. Thyrotoxicosis is a rare medical emergency.

A special mention must be made regarding heart failure from oncological diseases. Both chemotherapeutic agents, as well as modern therapy based on monoclonal antibodies, antienzymatic, antihormonal, can have negative effects on the myocardium with a decrease in EF and the onset of heart failure [8].

Thus, the oncological disease becomes a chronic condition well controlled under modern therapy, but patients lose their functional capacity as a result of the development of heart failure. In this sense, protocols have been established through which the oncological patients, under such cardiotoxic agents, enter the cardiological follow-up programs. Changes in FE are mainly monitored. Decreases of about 5% in these parameters require a change in oncological therapy. There are well known cases of patients, especially with hematological oncological diseases, who after 8-10 years of healing develop heart failure. That's why the cardio-oncology has become a frontier discipline, with involvement in the functional recovery of patients.

Heart failure is diagnosed clinically, based on signs and symptoms. Paraclinical tests only confirm the diagnosis and help establish the etiology.

That is why a correct evaluation of the functional capacity should be done with specific tests in this sense. The most relevant test is the cardiorespiratory exercise test. It uses an objective indicator of tissue perfusion, namely oxygen consumption (VO2) which is closely correlated with cardiac function. However, the cardio-respiratory exercise test is not currently used, but rather for research purposes.

Another very widespread test that also allows the evaluation of functional capacity is the exercise ECG test on the treadmill (or bicycle). In addition to data related to ischemia, the evolution of blood pressure and arrhythmias, it also estimates the level of energy consumed by the patient's metabolism.

It is expressed in METs (Metabolic Equivalent) and at rest has a value of 1. It is calculated according to age, weight, height. A value of > 7 recorded during exercise in the case of a patient with heart failure is considered that the respective patient has a good functional capacity with a risk of small cardiovascular complications. At a value < 5, the patient cannot perform medium or intense effort, and is considered to express a low functional capacity.

Diseases prevent the functioning of the individual, from a physical, mental, professional and social point of view, so they determine a functional deficit [3]. Affecting the individual on a social and professional level has a major implication, being able to generate a vicious circle with the involvement of psychological aspects (anxiety, depression) and worsening of the underlying problem [4,5].

Functional impairment is the consequence of morphological changes or varied functional disorders (diseases, accidents, genetic anomalies), it is quantifiable standardized through clinical and functional evaluations [9]. In the medical expertise in the cases of cardio-respiratory insufficiency, we use the NYHA functional classification scale, depending on the severity of dyspnea.

- NYHA class I – dyspnea occurs with very high efforts, without limitation of physical activity;
- NYHA class II – dyspnoea occurs at medium efforts, with minimal limitation of physical activity;
- NYHA class III – dyspnea occurs at low efforts, with a significant limitation of physical activity;
- NYHA Class IV – dyspnea occurs at rest with an inability to perform any physical activity.

and ejection fraction:

- Normal EF above 55%
- Mild systolic dysfunction FE=45-54%
- Moderate systolic dysfunction FE=30-44%
- Severe systolic dysfunction EF below 30% [3,6].

For objectification, a percentage calculation is used, made by fitting into a grid of criteria and norms, which vary for each insurance company/health insurance company/pension company. In fact, even in Romania, which has an advanced legislation compared to France, Sweden, Norway, we still have different criteria grids for the sickness pension and for obtaining the disabled person certificate, grids approved by legislation [10].

The patient with heart failure is also entitled to a disability certificate and disability pension, depending on the criteria in force in the country where he is applying for social insurance rights. The criteria are established by a working group made up of expert doctors and university professors in the respective field, are approved by law (in Romania) and are periodically re-evaluated, taking into account the guidelines proposed by the European professional associations [10].

Criteria Table

Functional Deficit		Work Capacity	Disability Degree
Patients with dyspnea on high efforts, PHT and mild RVH, AVB gr. I or gr. II type 1, RBBB, sinus node disease with asymptomatic bradycardia, mild systolic dysfunction	Easy 20-49%	Kept	It doesn't fit
Dyspnea on high and moderate exertion, moderate PHT and RVH, rare angina attacks, episodic rhythm disturbances, NYHA II, EF=40-44%	Medium 50-69%	Least half lost	Grade III
Dyspnea on low exertion, severe PHT, signs of right heart failure, EF=39-30%, NYHA III-IV with severe rhythm and/or conduction disturbances, intracavitary thrombosis, frequent anginal attacks that are difficult to respond to medication	Accentuated 70-89%	Totally lost	Grade II

Dyspnea on minimal exertion or with orthopnea, with signs of decompensated, irreversible right heart failure, anginal attacks at rest, EF below 30%, NYHA IV, severe ventricular arrhythmias with risk of sudden death, recurrent acute pulmonary edema	Serious 90-100%	Work capacity and self-service completely lost	Grade I

People with special needs (handicap) represent those people who have lasting deficiencies, which, in interaction with various barriers, can limit the equal participation of those people in society [12,15].

For disability, work capacity, we have four categories: mild, medium, accentuated and severe. For the severely disabled, we have two possibilities – with and without a companion [10,12].

The disability pension falls into 3 categories:

- Grade III the patient with medium functional deficit has the right to work part-time
- Grade II, the patient with a pronounced/accentuated functional deficit may work in limited conditions
- Grade I the patient with severe functional deficit, without self-service capacity, with a accompanying person, may work in limited conditions (for example blind people) [3,13].

Currently, only medical criteria are used to assess a patient claiming social security rights. All insurance expert doctors take into account the professional background of the patient at the time of assessment - you cannot expertise a ditch digger and a teacher in the same way, even if they both had a myocardial infarction with the same clinical signs.

From this point of view, I support the re-introduction of medico-social criteria grids (as they exist in the USA), because they will help expert doctors to better evaluate the work capacity of patients [14].

Cardiorespiratory failure is a difficult syndrome to assess due to the summation of contributing etiological factors, psychological impact and comorbidities. The patient who has this affliction will be examined patiently, gently, and will be asked what he wishes to do in the future. Many patients want to continue working. I can give two examples that impressed me, from my patients:

1. A young doctor, an anesthesiologist, preferred to work, although he was immobilized in a wheelchair.

2. A 60-year-old patient with stage III heart failure wanted to continue working as a block administrator in order to have money for medication.

The psychological, social and financial impact of retirement is very high and that is why in the last 15 years in Great Britain a great emphasis has been placed on return to work, RTW, return to work, an integrative concept, modern and old at the same time.

RTW is designed as a re-adaptation of patients to work, re-integration into the collective, recovery of working capacity (spa treatments, physiotherapy and physiotherapy, psychotherapy), offering a protected job, flexible or reduced schedule (4-6 hours/day).

The patient becomes a person with special needs who is socially integrated, instead of being a marginalized social worker.

Conclusions

The cardiorespiratory failure is a difficult syndrome to assess, due to the summation of the contributing etiological factors, the psychological impact and the comorbidities.

The patient, who has this affliction, will be examined patiently, gently, and will be asked what he/she wishes to do in the future.

Many patients want to continue working.

References

1. http://circ.ahajournals.org/content/105/11/1387.short, https://doi.org/10.1161/hc1102.105289 Circulation. 2002;105:1387-1393 Originally published March 19, 2002
2. Aurel Marin and all, Heart Failure, Etna Publishing House, 2017, ISBN 978-973-1795-23-7

3. http://onlinelibrary.wiley.com/doi/10.1016/j.ejheart.2008.08.005/full, ESC Guidelines for the diagnosis and treatment of acute and chronic heart failure 2008
4. Gabriele Masini, Fraser J. Graham, Pierpaolo Pellicori, John G.F. Cleland, Joseph J. Cuthbert, Syed Kazmi, Riccardo M. Inciardi, Andrew L. Clark; Criteria for Iron Deficiency in Patients with Heart Failure; JACC. 2022 Feb, 79 (4) 341–351
5. Andrew Xanthopoulos, Adamantia Papamichail, Alexandros Briasoulis, Konstantinos Loritis, Angeliki Bourazana, Dimitrios E. Magouliotis, Pantelis Sarafidis, Ioannis Stefanidis, John Skoularigis, and Filippos Triposkiadis; Heart Failure in Patients with Chronic Kidney Disease; J Clin Med. 2023 Sep; 12(18): 6105.
6. Marijana Tadic, Cesare Cuspidi, Francesca Calicchio, Guido Grassi, Giuseppe Mancia; Diabetic cardiomyopathy: How can cardiac magnetic resonance help?; Acta Diabetologica Volume 57, pages 1027–1034, (2020)
7. Kittleson MM, Ruberg FL, Ambardekar AV, et al.; 2023 ACC Expert Consensus Decision Pathway on Comprehensive Multidisciplinary Care for the Patient With Cardiac Amyloidosis; J Am Coll Cardiol 2023; Jan 23
8. Irwin Klein, MD, and Sara Danzi, PhD; Thyroid disease and the heart; https://doi.org/10.1161/CIRCULATIONAHA.106.67832
9. Michael Cronin and co; Heart Failure Association-International Cardio-Oncology Society Risk Score Validation in HER2-Positive Breast Cancer; J Clin Med 2023 Feb 6;12(4):1278. doi: 10.3390/jcm 12041278
10. Criteria and norms for clinical, functional diagnosis and assessment of work capacity, Annex to HG 1542/2022, MO nr. 1243 bis/22.12.2022, p 4-5
11. Pain Therapy, Publishing House Etna and Publishing House Viața medicală, 2017, pg 128
12. Soare Ioana, International Pensions – Insurance Medicine, Editura Etna, 2010
13. Mann Douglas L. Zipes Douglas P., Libby Peter, Bonow Robert O., Braunwald' s Heart Disease: A Textbook of Cardiovascular Medicine, 8th edition, Ed. Elsevier
14. L448/2006, low regarding protection and promotion of disabled persons rights, http://www.mmuncii.ro/pub/imagemanager/images/file/Legislatie/LEGI/L448-2006_rep.pdf, 01.08.2016

PART 7

REHABILITATION

CHAPTER 1

RETURN TO WORK

IOANA SOARE

Return to work (RTW) was imposed as a topic by social/ insurance medicine (Germany, UK, Romania).

It is defined as the process of integrating the patient into a work routine and a work environment after sick leave, is also one of the main predictive factors for a successful prognosis and evolution of the patient's initial impairment [1].

At European level, we study the factors determining return to work / RTW and the social determinants of disease retirement (loneliness, reduced education, rural housing with difficult access to medical services, age over 50, female sex, poverty, low wages). These factors were highlighted in very big studies - Framingham, Trondheim. The social factors have a greater impact on the evolution and prognosis, subsequently upon RTW, as the medical factors.

European Union of Medicine in Assurance and Social Security, EUMASS, proposed the following definitions:

Rehabilitation includes the set of measures that can be applied to persons with an impairment of their functional capacity due to ill-health, in order to integrate or reintegrate them into professional (RTW) and social activity [2].

RTW is an integrative concept implying:

- Work capacity recovery
- Medical rehabilitation (physical and psychological)
- Work place adaptation
- Working hours adaptation
- Readapting to work
- Avoiding stress situation and factors

- Programs for the inclusion in the work group
- Income restauration
- Social restauration [3].

and

- Discussions with the direct chief and the family members [4].

RTW is not Fit for work - the occupational doctor will consider each working place and each job, then the patient and will issue a Fit for work form, allowing or not the patient to work on a specific job.

Return to work may be initiated via two paths, starting with the physician's work release or with a proposal from the employer or a qualified rehabilitation professional. In either case, the release must be as specific as possible so the employer and patient clearly understand what is expected [5].

RTW depends upon:

- Multidisciplinary medical program
- Length of short-term sick leave
- Support at work
- Workplace intervention - adaptation, support in college relationships, low or flexible program [3,4,5,6].

The primary goal of all these measures is to help the patient to stay integrated, not to give up and retire [1].

Disability pension/benefit is seen by many patients as a solution to all their problems. Often, however, discontinuing professional activity and leaving the work group can and does frequently lead to a worsening of the symptomatology [1,6].

Following RTW the patient becomes a person with special needs, socially integrated [1].

The social determinants for return to work / RTW and for the invalidity pension (loneliness, reduced education, rural housing with difficult access to medical services, age over 50, female sex, poverty, low wages) are most important [1,5,6].

Examples

Patients who had TB have low chances to get employed [7].

Patients with COPD have less chances as the psychotic patients to return to work. They may profit from working, in terms of money, social wellbeing [8].

We must be attentive to patients with Obstructive Sleep Apnoea, a disease recognized more often now [9].

Multidisciplinary interventions involving physical, psycho-educational and/or vocational components led to higher RTW rates in patients with cancer [10,11].

Patients who have received lung transplants, after 6 months may return to work, if possible [12,13].

Conclusions

RTW is therapeutic.

Rehabilitation implies medical and social factors, and a qualified team.

References

1. Soare Ioana, Medical expertise, Insurance Medicine (Expertiză medicală, medicină de asigurări), ETNA Publishing House, 2017, p115.
2. Corina Oancea, Soren Brage, Freddy Falez, Wout de Boer, The role of the (social) insurance physician in vocational rehabilitation, An international survey, 2016. www.eumass.com.
3. van Vilsteren M, van Oostrom SH, de Vet HC, Franche RL, Boot CR, Anema JR., Workplace interventions to prevent work disability in workers on sick leave, Cochrane Database Syst Rev. 2015 Oct 5;(10):CD006955. doi: 10.1002/14651858.CD006955.pub3.
4. Adela Popa, Mihai Stelian Rusu, Felicia Morândău, Alexandra Sidor, Radu-Ioan Popa, Community participation for reducing the burden of cancer: stakeholders' involvement in facilitating the return to work of cancer patients, Romanian Ministry of Education, CNCS-UEFISCDI Project number PN-II-RU-TE-2014-4-0478 (contract no. 363 din

01/10/2015) Social Research Centre, University Lucian Blaga, Sibiu, Romania.
5. Williams Nerys, The British Approach to Vocational Rehabilitation, Romanian Journal of Insurance Medicine, vol 15, 1/2009, 5-7.
6. Popa AE, Bejenaru A, Mitrea EC, Morândău F, Pogan L. Return to work after chronic disease: A theoretical framework for understanding the worker-employer dynamic. Chronic Illness. August 2022. doi:10.1177/17423953221117852
7. Săftescu Sorin, Vidoni Livia, Return to work after invalidity pension, Romanian Journal of Insurance Medicine, vol.19, 4/2013, 19-25.
8. Oliver Christian Goehl, Training in COPD, ISBN 978-3-98-167146-9, Print Media Innovation, Hamburg, Germany, 62-63.
9. Sukwoo Hong, Yewon Kim, Ji-Young Ryu,[1] Sangyoon Lee,[1] Byung-Chul Son,[2] Chae-Kwan Lee,[2] and Dae-Hwan Kim, A case of obstructive sleep apnea and assessments of fitness for work, Ann Occup Environ Med. 2014; 26: 7. Published online 2014 Apr 25. doi: 10.1186/2052-4374-26-7, https://www.ncbi.nlm.nih.gov/pmc/articles/PMC4017773/. http://onlinelibrary.wiley.com/doi/10.1002/14651858.cd007569.pub3/full.
10. Kvillemo P, Mittendorfer-Rutz E, Bränström R, Nilsson K, Alexanderson K. Sickness Absence and Disability Pension After Breast Cancer Diagnosis: A 5-Year Nationwide Cohort Study. J Clin Oncol. 2017 Jun 20;35(18):2044-2052. doi: 10.1200/JCO.2015.66.0613. Epub 2017 May 1.
11. Angela Gem de Boer Tyna K Taskila, Seitske J Tamminga, Michael Feuerstein, Monique HW Frings-Dresen, Jos H Verbeek, Interventions to Enhance Return-to-Work for Cancer Patients,
12. De Baere C, Delva D, Kloeck A, Remans K, Vanrenterghem Y, Verleden G, Vanhaecke J, Nevens F, Dobbels F. Return to work and social participation: does type of organ transplantation matter? Transplantation. 2010 Apr 27;89(8):1009-15. doi: 10.1097/TP.0b013e3181ce77e5.
13. Hendrik Suhling, Christine Knuth, Axel Haverich, Heidrun Lingner, Tobias Welte, and Jens Gottlieb, Employment after Lung Transplantation—a Single-Center Cross-Sectional Study, Dtsch Arztebl Int. 2015 Mar; 112(13): 213–219, published online 2015 Mar 27. doi: 10.3238/arztebl.2015.0213.

CHAPTER 2

PULMONARY REHABILITATION OF PATIENTS WITH COPD: FROM THE BEGINNINGS TO THE 21ST CENTURY

PARASCHIVA POSTOLACHE AND ŞTEFAN SĂNDULACHE

> "Diet alone will not keep a man healthy; he must also exercise. Nutrition and exercise, although they have opposite effects, they also work together to generate health."
> —Hippocrates (460 – 377 BC)

As early as 1821, Laënnec (1771-1826), the inventor of the stethoscope, described the use of kinetotherapy in chest disorders [1].

Thomas Beddoes of Bristol established around 1800 an Institute for patients with heart disease and asthma.

Laënnec, Beddoes and Denison noted, almost two centuries ago, that exercise was an important element in the process of rehabilitation.

Exercise and any form of effort, 70-80 years ago, were considered avoidable in patients with pulmonary or heart diseases [2].

In the '70s and '80s, Pulmonary Rehabilitation (PR) pioneers [3] needed valid and reproducible evidence to combat the current skepticism, that PR did not produce any improvement in lung volumes and airflow limitation. Some studies in the 1980s questioned the efficacy of PR and so the field took a step backwards. Research with biochemical markers of exercise biopsies has not demonstrated a physiological effect of exercise in COPD patients.

However, researchers noted that other benefits, related to dyspnea and quality of life, were obtained as a result of PR, but they had no methods to quantify these improvements [4].

PR is very effective in reducing the systemic effects of chronic lung disease, such as peripheral muscle dysfunction caused by physical deconditioning.

The American Thoracic Society (ATS) published in 1981 an important paper, which showed an improvement of symptoms in patients undergoing PR procedures.

In 1982, Butland and collaborators evaluated the possibility of reducing the time patients would have to walk when tested to highlight the level of their physical condition. The subjects they studied showed reduced motivation to perform the 12 minutes of physical activity (based on the walking distance during the 12-minute test, described by Cooper as a guide to physical training in healthy young men), a test used in the military to measure the physical condition of recruits. Butland compared the 12-minute, 6-minute and 2-minute walk tests, and the 6-minute walk test correlated strongly with the 12-minute test [5]. The ATS standardized the 6-minute walk test (6MWT) in 2002 [6].

In 1987, Guyatt developed The Chronic Respiratory Questionnaire (CRQ), a questionnaire that assesses the effects of PR treatment on quality of life in clinical trials and is currently available in 45 languages [7].

The importance of PR has returned to attention in the '90s. American universities began offering postgraduate courses in cardiopulmonary rehabilitation. A. Ries summarized in 1990 knowledge and scientific basis in a systematic review [8]. Ries and his colleagues at University of California, San Diego, published the first randomized, controlled study to evaluate the effects of PR over 6 years and compare the effects of a comprehensive PR program with those of the education alone [9].

The year 1992 marked the creation of Saint George's Respiratory Questionnaire (SGRQ), conducted by Johns in the UK. The questionnaire is widely used in COPD, but is validated for use in bronchiectasis, kyphoscoliosis and sarcoidosis. The author concluded that the SGRQ is a valid means of assessing health status in chronic diseases with airflow limitation [10]. The same team, led by Jones, developed in 2009 COPD Assessment Test (CAT), which is the new questionnaire for people with COPD, now available online in 57 languages [11].

In the new millennium, new studies have been conducted and scientific information about PR has been extended to patients with other chronic lung diseases besides COPD and adjuvant exercise methods have been tested. Trooster has investigated the benefits of rehabilitation programs, demonstrating that the benefits are greater the longer the program [12].

The US National Heart, Lung and Blood Institute (NHLBI), in collaboration with the World Health Organization (WHO), launched the Global Initiative for Chronic Obstructive Lung Disease (GOLD) in 1998 to raise awareness of COPD and to help patients with the condition who may die prematurely from COPD or its complications [13]. The GOLD Consensus "Global Strategy for the Diagnosis, Management and Prevention of COPD" was published in 2001 and immediately after its publication a network of international experts (GOLD National Leaders) worked to implement the report's recommendation, that PR is the gold standard of care for COPD patients.

Lately, various guidelines and manuals address the topic of PR, which help guide healthcare providers in this satisfying field. For example, on Medline in 1990 there were 500 citations on COPD and the number has grown to more than 3,000 by 2010.

According to GOLD 2022, COPD " is a common, preventable, and treatable disease that is characterized by persistent respiratory symptoms and airflow limitation that is due to airway and/or alveolar abnormalities usually caused by significant exposure to noxious particles or gases and influenced by host factors including abnormal lung development" [14]. It has become the 3rd leading cause of death globally and 8th on the Disability Adjusted Life Years (DALY) scale.

For a comprehensive approach to disease management, the importance of non-pharmacological treatment, which must be complementary to pharmacological therapy, has also been highlighted [15].

Pulmonary rehabilitation treatment is central to these patients and is recognized by all specialists in the field. The current definition of PR, following the Official American Thoracic Society Workshop Report published in May 2021, is based on definitions previously developed, based on scientific evidence, by pulmonary rehabilitation specialists, which have been published since 1974 and updated in 2006, 2007, 2013 and 2015. According to this report, "Pulmonary rehabilitation is a comprehensive intervention based on a thorough patient assessment followed by patient-tailored therapies that include, but are not limited to, exercise training, education, and behavior change, designed to improve the physical and psychological condition of people with chronic respiratory disease and to promote the long-term adherence to health-enhancing behaviors" [16].

Pulmonary rehabilitation with its core components, including physical training combined with disease-specific education, improves exercise capacity, symptoms and quality of life **in all grades of COPD severity**, and is essential for COPD patients as early as stage II (GOLD B), with physical activity recommended from stage I (GOLD A). Rehabilitation programs should begin in the hospital (in - patient program), with maintenance and home practice of techniques learned in the hospital, with periodic return to the hospital for further sessions (out - patient program). The duration of a programme is a minimum of 6 to 8 weeks, with periodic return to hospital, aiming at the patient learning a new lifestyle (avoidance of risk factors, daily physical activity as long as possible, in which the new breathing pattern becomes a reflex stereotype, practicing energy conservation strategies) [17].

A PR programme, given good patient adherence, is successful if:

- a "braking" of the decline in lung function was achieved;
- an increase in exercise capacity was achieved (e.g. the 6-minute walk test improved by 10-25% or the feeling of dyspnoea during exercise was reduced);
- improved quality of life through increased independence in carrying out daily activities;
- reduced feelings of breathlessness, depression and/or anxiety;
- reduced number or severity of exacerbations [**18**].

The positive effects of PR are also visible in the presence of abnormalities in lung architecture, due to the fact that many of the disabilities arise through systemic effects of chronic respiratory conditions (hypoxaemia, wasting, decreased muscle mass, depression, isolation) and comorbidities (cardiovascular disease, osteoporosis, depression, diabetes, obesity). The PR program is individualized, not universally applicable for every patient [**19**], and the PR team consists of (Fig. 1):

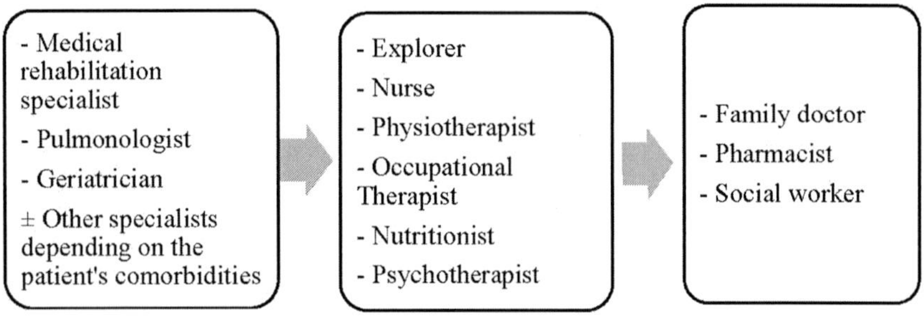
- Medical rehabilitation specialist
- Pulmonologist
- Geriatrician
± Other specialists depending on the patient's comorbidities
- Explorer
- Nurse
- Physiotherapist
- Occupational Therapist
- Nutritionist
- Psychotherapist
- Family doctor
- Pharmacist
- Social worker

Figure 1. The team involved in pulmonary rehabilitation [**20**]

The components of the PR programme (fig. 2) are the following:

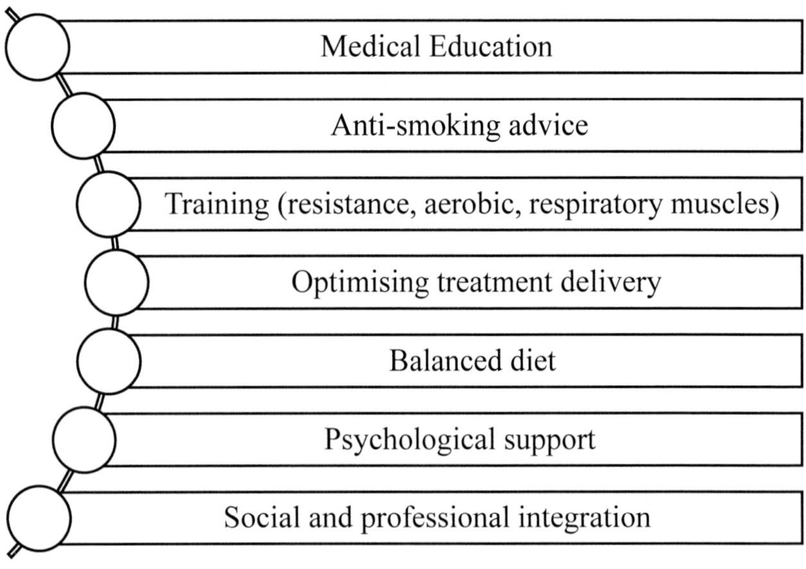

Figure 2. The components of the PR programme [21]

Medical education is an effective and inexpensive method that increases the patient's confidence in their own strength to fight their illness and their trust in all those around them in their generous attempt to alleviate suffering and improve quality of life. Medical education is ongoing, beginning at the first consultation and continuing throughout the patient's follow-up. Educational support has always been considered a key feature in the management of patients with respiratory disease [22]. In one study, Brandsetter et al. showed that only 34% of patients with COPD were fully adherent to drug treatment. Non-adherence to pharmacological treatment could be multifactorial, in most cases patients underestimating symptoms and not being fully aware of their disease and therefore not understanding the importance of medication administration. In addition, as for other respiratory diseases, treatment relies on inhalation of medication from different devices, which requires patient collaboration for correct medication administration [23].

Dosed physical training is one of the most important components of physiotherapy and PR programs. The exercise program is individualized for each patient according to: disease severity, age, gender, associated diseases, training methods (Table 1, 2), duration, pace, intensity of effort, motivation and patient choice [24].

Exercises will address different muscle groups: to increase the endurance of the lower limb muscles, walking on a treadmill, pedalling on a cycle ergometer, counteracting some weights (exercises should also be performed by people sitting or lying down to move the limbs, increase flexibility and decrease joint stiffness), as well as stretching, coordination and attention exercises; to increase endurance of upper limb muscles, weights or stretching exercises are recommended; for trunk muscles, stretching gymnastics, swimming, cycling, treadmill; neck and head gymnastics, breathing techniques (abdominal breathing) [25].

The cycloergometer is a device used for both diagnosis (cardiopulmonary exercise testing) and treatment (training) (Fig. 3).

Table 1. Types of training used in PR [26]

Aerobic training - improves exercise capacity and endurance time			
Type of exercise	Intensity	Duration	Frequency
Walking	- 80% of the average speed of 6MWT - 60 - 70% of maximum heart rate at 6MWT - BORG scale 3 - 4 (moderate)	20 – 30 minutes	4 – 5 sessions per week
Treadmill	- 80% of the average speed of 6MWT - 60 - 70% of maximum heart rate at 6MWT - BORG scale 3 - 4 (moderate) - speed reduction by 0.5 - 1 km/hour until familiar with treadmill	20 – 30 minutes	4 – 5 sessions per week
Cycling	- BORG scale 3 – 4 (moderate)	20 – 30 minutes	4 – 5 sessions per week

Table 2. Types of training used in PR [27]

Resistance training – improves muscle force and resistance		
Type of exercise	Intensity	Frequency
For upper limbs - **Dumbbell push-ups** - **Pull-ups** - **Chest press**	- 1 set = 10 repetitions - BORG scale 2 – 3 (mild or moderate)	- 2 – 3 sessions per week - At least 1 day in between sessions
For lower limbs - **Genoflexions** - **Climbing stairs** - **Elastic bands**	- 1 set = 10 repetitions - BORG scale 2 – 3 (mild or moderate)	- 2 – 3 sessions per week - At least 1 day in between sessions

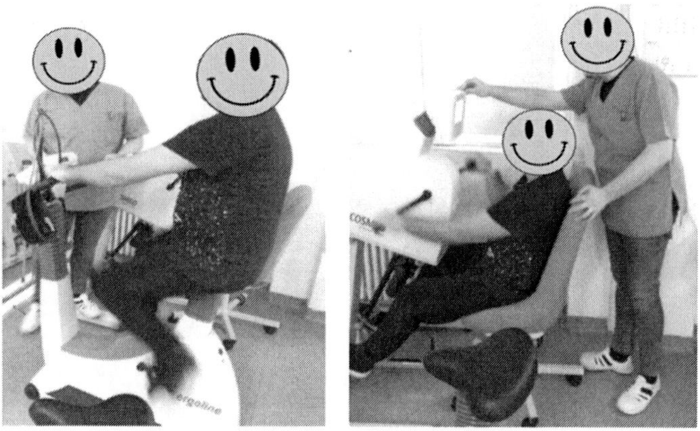

Figure 3. Dosed exercise training with cycloergometer for lower and upper body. [Photo source: Respiratory Rehabilitation Clinic, Rehabilitation Clinical Hospital, Iasi, Romania; Head of Clinical Section: Assoc. Prof. Paraschiva POSTOLACHE, M.D., Ph.D]

Respiratory muscle training

Respiratory muscle training (RMT) is a valuable method that provides additional PR benefits by improving both muscle strength and endurance with clinical benefits in COPD patients who remain symptomatic despite optimal therapy [27]. The aim of RMT is to improve respiratory muscle function, hypoxia, hypoventilation and dyspnea relief [28].

RMT involves the training of inspiratory and expiratory muscles. Depending on the type of exercise, training can be forceful, consisting of repeated series of breaths with increased resistance, or endurance (forced ventilation maintained for several minutes). In general, **inspiratory muscle training** is used in patients with dyspnea as the predominant symptom, and **expiratory muscle training** in patients with productive cough [29].

Before starting the training program, the maximal inspiratory pressure in the oral cavity (Fig. 4), which represents the inspiratory muscle exercise capacity, should be assessed, as the methods and equipment used for the two types of training differ significantly [30].

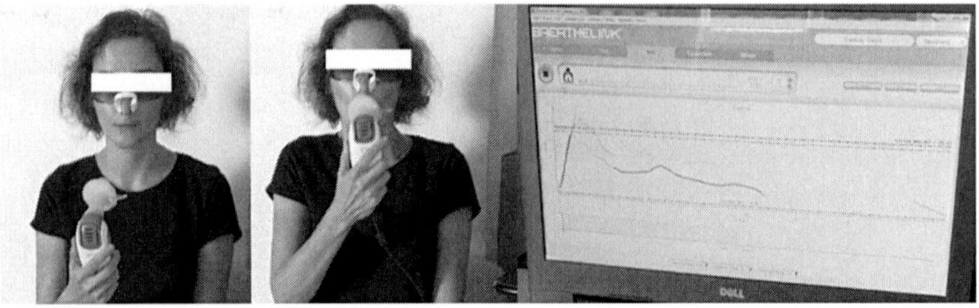

Figure 4. Respiratory muscle pressure testing. [Photo source: Respiratory Rehabilitation Clinic, Rehabilitation Clinical Hospital, Iasi, Romania; Head of Clinical Section: Assoc. Prof. Paraschiva POSTOLACHE, M.D., Ph.D]

Endurance training, achieved by maintaining forced hyperventilation for several minutes, trains both the inspiratory and expiratory muscles. In this type of training, the respiratory muscles are forced to work at high speeds over a prolonged period of time. For training based on increasing muscle strength, devices are used that impose increased resistance on the oral cavity, with the muscles being subjected to an increased external load.

Various devices are used for RMT, including the stimulation spirometer, Pflex resistance breathing, flutter valve and Threshold inspiratory valve breathing.

The stimulation spirometer (fig. 5) is a device containing several balls, which rise according to the strength of the respiratory flow. During this training, the patient must generate a target inspiratory-expiratory flow, which propels the beads to the top of the device. As the breathing capacity increases, the balls rise higher. The advantage of this device is that it provides encouraging visual feedback to the patient [31].

Breathing against a Pflex resistance is a workout consisting of a series of repeated exhalations and inhalations against an increased resistance given by a fixed diameter hole on the inspiratory circuit with six levels of resistance. This technique is dependent on respiratory flow and sessions of 10 - 15 minutes per day are recommended throughout the PR program.

Threshold training (fig. 5) allows a load to be applied at a variable, quantifiable intensity, the pressure being easily adjusted by simply rotating the distal end of the device. Threshold loading benefits inspiratory muscle strength. The device has an adjustable resistance level from 7 to 41 cm H2O. Patients will train with this device for 30 minutes daily at a resistance of 30 to 60% of the initial value of the maximum inspiratory pressure in the oral cavity. In one study, a group of researchers demonstrated the superiority of the Threshold device compared to the stimulation spirometer [32].

Isocapnic ventilation training - also called endurance training - is a technique that consists of forced ventilation at high flow rates sustained over several minutes. To train the inspiratory muscles, patients will breathe in through a device, usually the POWERBreathe, which imposes a resistance equivalent to 30-60% of the initial maximum inspiratory pressure at the level of the oral cavity (Fig. 5). Exercises will be performed for 30 minutes daily, in sessions of three to five minutes, with a two-minute break between sessions, at home or in special PR centres, increasing the resistance of the device by 5% per week. Isocapnic hyperpnea is a physically demanding method that requires a high degree of commitment and motivation from the patient. The POWERBreathe device contains an inhalation resistance valve. The exercises depend on the patient's tolerance and the degree of respiratory failure. RMT should be performed daily and continued throughout life to maintain beneficial effects.

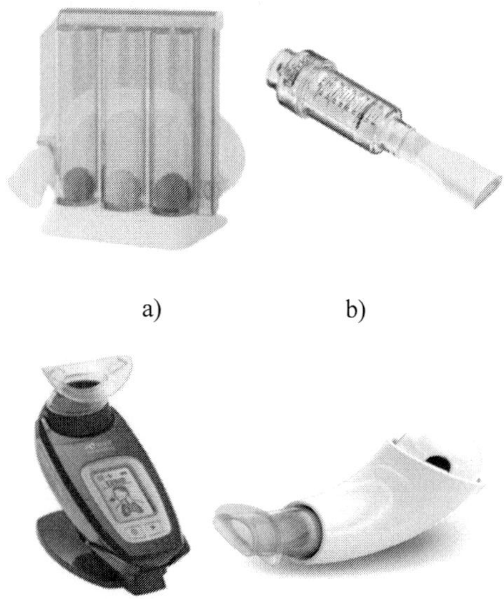

a) b)

c) d)

Figure 5. Devices for Respiratory Muscle Training. Stimulation spirometer; b) Threshold; c) POWERBreathe; d) Shaker Plus. [Photo source: Respiratory Rehabilitation Clinic, Rehabilitation Clinical Hospital, Iasi, Romania; Head of Clinical Section: Assoc. Prof. Paraschiva POSTOLACHE]

The Threshhold PEP Expiratory Muscle Trainer has the same one-way flow valve system, which opens as the patient exhales, creating positive pressure that keeps the airway open and allows bronchial secretions to escape during coughing. It has an adjustable resistance level from 4 to 20 cm H_2O. The most widely used device for training expiratory muscles is the Shaker Plus (Fig. 5, 6) [33].

According to international guidelines, RMT should be continued after patients are discharged from PR centers on a daily basis, on its own, or, associated with the PR program, a program that can be carried out at home, or if possible, in specialized PR centers, at least two to three times a week, to maintain the effects of the training [34].

The largest group of patients enrolled in the PR program are with COPD, but also with other chronic lung diseases, and for COPD patients there is sufficient evidence that PR improves daily symptoms, exercise capacity, quality of life and health status, independent of the stage and complexity of the disease. An ongoing PR program, which includes exercise training, education, and other interventions, is safe and has benefits for most patients with chronic lung disease [35].

Since 2001, the Global Obstructive Lung Disease Initiative declared PR as a standard of care for people with COPD. There are still unresolved issues and information gaps that require specialist attention [36].

For COPD patients, recent studies have also identified different subgroups of patients based on key disease characteristics such as lung function, physical activity, body composition and comorbidities. However, **identification of COPD phenotypes is still necessary**, and longitudinal studies need to validate the utility of established phenotypes and explore sources of variability in phenotypes and temporal nature. Most studies are cross-sectional and have shown that it is possible to discriminate between groups with similar characteristics, but there is still a lack of data on whether such phenotypes are associated with long-term outcomes or response to classical or personalized PR [Franssen F et al., 2019]. Because chronic respiratory diseases are typically complex and heterogeneous, stratifying patients into groups that share similar treatable traits is important for optimizing the effectiveness of patient management [37].

The last four years have presented us with a new challenge: telemedicine, which is defined by the World Health Organization as “the provision of healthcare services, where distance is a critical factor, by all health professionals, through the use of information technologies and communication for the exchange of valid information for the diagnosis, treatment and prevention of diseases and injuries", in which respiratory telerehabilitation (Table 1) occupies an important place [38]

Table 1. Respiratory telerehabilitation: advantages and disadvantages [39, 40, 41, 42]

Advantages	Disadvantages
• The patient is in the family environment; • Allows the patient to be autonomous, confident; • The recovery process is facilitated and a real acceleration can be observed; • Telemedicine / telerehabilitation removes geographical and distance barriers; • Everything can take place on secure medical communication platforms, where data confidentiality is strictly maintained; • Reduce healthcare costs; • Saving the time needed to travel home; • Wider access to the PR program; • The PR program can be monitored;	• Patients need to know the technology; • Requires internet connection; • Inability to perform the PR program without the presence of a qualified and trained medical staff for what it means to assist in respiratory rehabilitation; • There is currently no legal framework in Romania to regulate the activity of telemedicine; • Lack of transparency regarding data security; • Lack of information and trust in specific eHealth solutions among patients, citizens and healthcare professionals.

Telerehabilitation at home is a useful option for patients who are in the period after an acute illness and cannot be taken over by the recovery centers, but need to start the rehabilitation program as soon as possible. Although respiratory rehabilitation is a well-established therapeutic method, with proven benefits, 8 – 40 % of patients referred to hospital PR programs do not adhere to them, while 10 – 30 % of those who start the program do not complete it.

Telerehabilitation is a therapeutic tool that can be used successfully. There are studies comparing telerehabilitation with standard rehabilitation. They have shown favorable results in increasing respiratory capacity and reducing symptoms, as well as improving the quality of life of patients [43].

Telemedicine has proved its worth in the midst of the pandemic, when health and distance rules made it inaccessible for patients to participate in rehabilitation programs, including patients with SARS-CoV-2 infection, both in the acute phase and in the phase post-COVID-19, manifested predominantly by respiratory symptoms of rest and exertion, for which PR is required. In this context, telerehabilitation has been an extremely important aid. It has been used successfully in Wuhan hospitals, where patients with COVID-19, isolated in wards, have been given, through a telephone application, models of aerobic exercise, resistance training with elastic bands, and exercises for training the respiratory muscles, in the form of videos or written recommendations. The exercises were also recorded, the application also having a symptom monitoring system, which was transmitted from patients to doctors.

In a multicenter study conducted in Australia, which assessed the access of patients with chronic pulmonary diseases to technology, out of 254 participants, 92% had access to at least one electronic device, 70% a tablet or a computer and 85% a mobile phone, 60% of patients were willing to access telerehabilitation [44].

Technologies used to perform respiratory telerehabilitation include: home video conferencing, the use of smartphones, tablets, web platforms and pedometers connected to the internet, virtual reality and augmented reality. Progress in telemedicine focuses on augmented reality, which is based on the concept of real-time, barrier-free interaction. Augmented reality differs from virtual reality by creating a real-time physical environment using four computer-generated sensory inputs (sound, video, graphics, or GPS data), while virtual reality detaches contact from reality. The future of medicine is geared towards augmented reality, although there is currently very little evidence of its use in rehabilitation [45, 50].

The use of technologies provides patients with chronic respiratory diseases with extensive access to respiratory rehabilitation. The technological devices are multiple and can be used singly or combined, they being in a permanent development [46, 47, 48, 49].

In conclusion, the history of pumonary rehabilitation is interesting. What appeared to be an area or uncertainty, with obscure benefits, is now supported by evidence classified by experts as of the highest standard. It is also hoped that the coming years will provide even newer and more exciting ways for a wider and more important role of PR as a futuristic version of the field. With new, exciting and well-designed studies in adjuvant PR such as integrated care, early rehabilitation, rehabilitation beyond COPD, etc., this new discipline continues to grow!

References

1. Carlin BW. Pulmonary Rehabilitation: An Historical Perspective. Semin Respir Crit Care Med. 2009; 30: 629-635.
2. Berra K. Cardiac and pulmonary rehabilitation: historical perspectives and future needs. J Cardio-Pulm Rehab. 1991; 11: 8–11.
3. Intersociety Commission on Heart Disease. Pulmonary rehabilitation Study Group. Community resources for rehabilitation of patients with chronic obstructive pulmonary disease and cor pulmonale. Circulation. 1974; 49 (suppl 1): A1-A20.
4. Belman MJ, Kendregan BA. Exercise training fails to increase skeletal muscle enzymes in patients with chronic obstructive pulmonary disease. Am Rev Respir Dis. 1981; 123: 256-261.
5. Butland RJ, Pang J, Gross ER, et al. Two-, six-, and 12-minute walking tests in respiratory diseases. Br Med J. 1982; 284: 1607-1608.
6. ATS Statement guidelines for the 6-minute walking test. ATS Committee on Proficiency Standards for Clinical Pulmonary Function Laboratories. Am J Respir Crit Care Med. 2002; 166(1): 111-118.
7. Guyatt GH, Berman LB, Towsend M, et al. A measure of quality of life for clinical trials in chronic lung disease. Thorax. 1987; 42: 773-778.
8. Ries AL. Position paper of the American Association of Cardiovascular and Pulmonary rehabilitation: scientific basis of pulmonary rehabilitation. J Cardio-Pulm Rehab. 1990; 10: 418-441.
9. Ries AL. Prospective on pulmonary rehabilitation. J Cardio-Pulm Rehab. 2003; 23: 78-83.
10. Jones PW, Quirk FH, Baveystock CM, et al. A self-complete measure of health status for chronic airflow limitation. The St. Goerge's Respiratory Questionnaire. Am Rev Respir Dis. 1992; 145(6): 1321-1327.
11. Jones PW, Harding G, Berry P, Wiklund I, Chen WH, et al. Development and first validation of the COPD Assessment Test. Eur Respir J. 2009; 34: 648–654.
12. Trooster T, Gosselink R, Decramer M. Short and long –term effects of outpatient rehabilitation in patients with chronic obstructive pulmonary

didsease: a randomized trial. Am J Med. 2000 Aug 15; 109(3): 2012-2017.

13. Global initiative for Chronic Obstructive Lung Disease. Global Strategy for the diagnosis, management and prevention of chronic obstructive lung disease (GOLD). Available from: http://goldcopd.org/ [Accesed 22 July 2022].
14. Global Initiative for Chronic Obstructive Lung Disease 2022 Report. Available from: https://goldcopd.org/2022-gold-reports/. [Accesed 22 July 2022].
15. Postolache AP, Marciniuk DD. Handbook of Pulmonary Rehabilitation. New York: Nova Science Publishers, Inc., 2021.
16. Postolache AP. Tratat de Recuperare respiratorie. București: Editura ETNA, 2022.
17. Holland E, Cox N, Houchen-Wolloff L, et al. Defining Modern Pulmonary Rehabilitation an Official American Thoracic Society Workshop Report. Ann Am Thorac Soc. 2021 May; 18 (5): e12–e29.
18. Spruit MA, Wouters FM. Organizational aspects of pulmonary rehabilitation in chronic respiratory diseases. Respirology. 2019; 24:838–843.
19. Nici L, Donner C, Wouters E, et al. American Thoracic Society/European Respiratory Society statement on pulmonary rehabilitation. Am J Respir Crit Care Med. 2006 Jun 15; 173(12): 1390-413.
20. Spruit MA, Singh SJ, Garvey C, et. al. An Official American Thoracic Society/European Respiratory Society Statement: Key Concepts and Advances in Pulmonary Rehabilitation. Am J Respir Crit Care Med. 2013; 188(8): e13–e64, DOI: 10.1164/rccm.201309-1634ST, www.atsjournals.org.
21. Rochester C, Vogiatzis I, Holland A, et al. An Official American Thoracic Society/European Respiratory Society Policy Statement: Enhancing Implementation, Use, and Delivery of Pulmonary Rehabilitation. Am J Respir Crit Care Med. 2015; 192(11): 1373–1386.
22. Donner C, Ambronsino N, Goldstein R. Pulmonary rehabilitation. New York: CRC Press, 2021.
23. Sami R, Saleni K, Hashemi M, et al. Exploring the barriers to pulmonary rehabilitation for patients with chronic obstructive pulmonary disease: a qualitative study. BMC Health Services Research 2021; 21:828-834.
24. Postolache AP, Cojocaru DC. Pulmonary Rehabilitation - from guidelines to practice. Rev Med Chir Soc Med Nat Iasi. 2013; 117(2): 380-387.

25. McSweeny AJ, Grant I, Heaton RK et al. Life quality of patients with chronic obstructive pulmonary disease. Arch Intern Med. 1982 Mar; 142(3):473-8.
26. Janjua S, Pike C, Carr R, et al. Interventions to improve adherence to pharmacological therapy for chronic obstructive pulmonary disease (COPD). Cochrane Database Syst Rev. 2019 Aug; 2019(8): CD013381.
27. Brandsetter S, Finger T, Fischer W, et al. Differences in medication adherence are associated with beliefs about medicines in asthma and COPD. Clin Transl Allergy. 2017; 7:39.
28. He GX, Li N, Ren L, et al. Benefits of different intensities of pulmonary rehabilitation for patients with moderate-to-severe COPD according to the GOLD stage: a prospective, multicenter, single-blinded, randomized, controlled trial. Int J Chron Obstruct Pulmon Dis. 2019; 14: 2291–2304.
29. Postolache AP, Meca AD. Exercise Program and Prescrioption in Pulmonary Reabilitation. In: Postolache AP, Marciniuk DD editors. Handbook of Pulmonary Rehabilitation. New York: Nova Science Publishers, Inc. 2021, 141-161.
30. Lung Foundation Australia. Pulmonary Reabilitation. Available from: https://pulmonaryrehab.com.au/importance-of-exercise/exercise-prescription-table/ [Accesed 22 October 2021].
31. Chen L, Su J. Pulmonary Rehabilitation Exercise Assessments and Training Methods for Patients with COPD: A Literature Review. Journal of Rehabilitation Therapy 2021 June; 3(1): 13-20.
32. Gloeck R, Schneeberger T, Jarosch I, et al. Pulmonary Rehabilitation and Exercise Training in Chronic Obstructive Pulmonary Disease. Dtsch Arztebl Int. 2019 Feb; 115(8): 117–123.
33. Chen H, Li P, Li N, et al. Rehabilitation effects of land and water-based aerobic exercise on lung function, dyspnea, and exercise capacity in patients with chronic obstructive pulmonary disease. Medicine (Baltimore). 2021 Aug 20; 100(33): e26976.
34. Zeng Y, Jiang F, Chen Y, et al. Exercise assessments and trainings of pulmonary rehabilitation in COPD: a literature review. Int J Chron Obstruct Pulmon Dis. 2018; 13: 2013-2023.
35. Postolache AP, Jimborean G, Ianoși ES, et al. Respiratory muscle training in chronic obstructive pulmonary disease. Pneumologia. 2017; 66(3): 128-131.
36. Hollebeke M, Gosselink R, Langer D. Training Specificity of Inspiratory Muscle Training Methods: a randomized trial. Front Physiol. 2020; 11: 1-13.

37. Gohl OC. Respiratory Muscle Training - Practical Aspects. In: Postolache AP, Marciniuk DD editors. Handbook of Pulmonary Rehabilitation. New York: Nova Science Publishers, Inc. 2021, 181-192.
38. Jimborean G, Ianoşi ES, Postolache AP. Respiratory Rehabilitation and Respiratory Muscle Training. In: Postolache AP, Marciniuk DD editors. Handbook of Pulmonary Rehabilitation. New York: Nova Science Publishers, Inc. 2021, 163-179.
39. Paiva DN, Assmann LB, Bordin DF, et al. Inspiratory muscle training with threshold or incentive spirometry: Which is the most effective? Rev Port Pneumol. 2015; 21(2): 76-81.
40. Garcia R. Pulmonary Rehabilitation: Time for an Upgrade. J Clin Med. 2020 Aug; 9(9):2742.
41. Franssen F, Alter P, Bar N, et al. Personalized medicine for patients with COPD: where are we? Int J Chron Obstruct Pulmon Dis. 2019; 14: 1465–1484.
42. Rochester C, Spruit M, Holland A. Pulmonary Rehabilitation in 2021. JAMA. 2021 Sep 14; 326(10): 969-970.
43. World Health Organization. Telemedicine: opportunities and developments in Member States: report on the second global survey on eHealth 2009. Available from: https://www.who.int/goe/publications/goe_telemedicine_2010.pdf [Accessed 7 April 2024].
44. Grigoletto I, Cavalheri V, de Lima F, et al. Recovery after COVID-19: The potential role of pulmonary rehabilitation. Braz J Phys Ther. 2020 Dec; 24(6): 463–464.
45. Stafinski T, Nagase FI, Avdagovska M, et al. Effectiveness of home-based pulmonary rehabilitation programs for patients with chronic obstructive pulmonary disease (COPD): systematic review. BMC Health Serv Res. 2022 Apr; 22(1):557.
46. Holland AE, Malaguti C, Hoffman M, et al. Home-based or remote exercise testing in chronic respiratory disease, during the COVID-19 pandemic and beyond: a rapid review. Chron Respir Dis. 2020 Dec; 17:1479973120952418.
47. Seidman Z, McNamara R, Wooton S, et al. People attending pulmonary rehabilitation demonstrate a substantial engagement with technology and willingness to use telerehabilitation: a survey. J Physiother. 2017 Jul; 63(3):175-181.
48. Colombo V, Aliverti A, Sacco M. Virtual reality for COPD rehabilitation: a technological perspective. Pulmonology 2020 Dec; S2531-0437(20) 30257-9. doi: 10.1016/j.pulmoe.2020.11.010.

49. Havot M, Saev D, Costes F, et al. Respiratory telerehabilitation in cases of COPD. Rev Mal Respir. 2022 Jan; S0761-8425(21): 00437-X.
50. Postolache AP. Tratat de Recuperare Respiratorie - aspecte particulare. Iaşi: Editura Gr. T. Popa, 2023.

CHAPTER 3

REHABILITATION FOR VISUALLY IMPAIRED PEOPLE

IOANA SOARE, SUHER ABDURAHMAN AND LAURA BATIS

Introduction

Individuals with disabilities (currently referred to as people with special needs) are those who have long-term physical, mental, intellectual, or sensory impairments, which, in interaction with various barriers, may hinder their full and effective participation in society on an equal basis with others [1, 2]. Visually impaired people, encompassing those with partial sight loss or complete blindness, experience the world in ways that often rely on non-visual senses such as hearing, touch, and smell. Despite challenges, many visually impaired individuals lead independent and fulfilling lives, aided by assistive technologies like screen readers, Braille displays, and voice-command devices. These tools, along with mobility aids like guide dogs or canes, help navigate daily tasks and environments. Inclusive design and accessibility are key to empowering visually impaired people, allowing them to engage fully with society, education, and employment. Moreover, awareness and understanding from the broader community can significantly enhance their quality of life, promoting greater inclusivity [3, 4].

Braille Era

A major milestone in assistive technology occurred in 1824 when Louis Braille invented the Braille system. Having lost his sight as a child, Louis developed this tactile writing method, using raised dots to symbolize letters and numbers. This innovation enabled blind individuals to read and write on their own, significantly transforming education and communication for the visually impaired. The Braille system has been successfully integrated into computer programs, enhancing accessibility for visually impaired users in the digital age. Specialized software and hardware, such as Braille displays and screen readers, convert digital text into Braille, allowing users to interact with computers more effectively. A Braille display connects to the computer and translates on-screen text into tactile Braille, which users can read line by line. Many operating systems and applications now include compatibility features for Braille, supporting the integration of assistive technologies that facilitate web browsing, document editing, and communication. This digital adaptation of the Braille system has significantly expanded opportunities for independence, education, and employment for blind individuals [4, 5].

Computers and AI

Computer programs designed for visually impaired people play a vital role in enhancing accessibility and independence in the digital world. These programs are tailored to overcome visual barriers by offering features like screen readers, which convert on-screen text into speech, and magnification tools that enlarge text and images. Some software even provides Braille display compatibility or voice-command functions, allowing users to interact with their devices using auditory cues. By breaking down the barriers posed by traditional visual interfaces, these assistive technologies enable visually impaired individuals to navigate the internet, work with documents, and engage in educational or professional activities with greater ease and efficiency [4].

The history of computer programs for visually impaired people traces back to the development of assistive technologies aimed at making computers accessible to those with vision impairments. In the early days of computing, accessibility was limited, but as personal computers gained prominence in the 1970s and 1980s, there was growing recognition of the need for tools that could make digital interfaces usable by everyone. One of the earliest breakthroughs was the development of screen readers in the 1980s, notably "OutSpoken" for the Apple Macintosh and "Job Access With Speech" (JAWS) for DOS in 1989. These programs allowed visually impaired users to listen to text on their screens by converting it to synthesized speech. Around the same time, Braille displays, which converted digital text into Braille, also emerged, further empowering blind users to engage with computers. Throughout the 1990s and 2000s, as graphical user interfaces (GUIs) became the norm, screen readers evolved to interpret these more complex visual environments. Companies like Microsoft and Apple began building accessibility features directly into their operating systems, with

Microsoft's "Windows Narrator" and Apple's "VoiceOver" becoming integral tools for accessibility [4].

In the modern era, technological advancements such as voice-command software, AI-driven screen readers, and mobile accessibility apps have expanded the capabilities of visually impaired individuals. These tools not only make computers more accessible but also open up the broader digital world, enabling people with visual impairments to engage in education, work, and social activities more independently and effectively than ever before. AI programs have significantly enhanced support for visually impaired individuals, empowering them with greater independence and accessibility. These programs use machine learning and computer vision to interpret the world through cameras or sensors, converting visual information into auditory descriptions or tactile feedback. For example, AI-driven apps can recognize objects, read text aloud, and identify faces, allowing users to navigate environments, read independently, and communicate more effectively. Advanced AI algorithms can even recognize currency, interpret colors, and offer scene descriptions, providing real-time information tailored to the user's surroundings. Popular devices like OrCam and apps such as Microsoft's Seeing AI make use of these technologies, promoting greater inclusivity by helping users participate more fully in daily life, education, and employment. By continuously learning and adapting to new contexts, these AI tools bring valuable enhancements to low-vision aids, making them more effective, responsive, and user-friendly [6, 7].

Modern glasses that utilize virtual reality (VR) and artificial intelligence (AI) are revolutionizing the way visually impaired individuals interact with their surroundings. These high-tech eyewear devices incorporate advanced features like real-time object recognition, text-to-speech capabilities, and augmented reality overlays to provide users with detailed descriptions of their environment. By processing visual information through AI algorithms, these glasses can identify faces, read signs, and even detect obstacles, delivering auditory or haptic feedback to guide users safely. Some models are designed to adapt to various lighting conditions, enhancing visibility in challenging environments. With their innovative approach, these smart glasses not only improve navigation and accessibility but also empower users to engage more confidently in daily activities, fostering greater independence and quality of life for those with visual impairments.

The OrCam MyEye, commonly referred to as OrCam, is a modern addition to the range of commercially available low-vision aids (LVAs). This portable device, which attaches to a user's eyeglass frame, includes a small camera that uses optical character recognition technology to convert printed or digital text into real-time audio feedback. Its primary users are individuals with severe visual impairments or blindness who are unable to read independently. Beyond text-to-speech, the OrCam also provides color, object, barcode, currency, and facial recognition capabilities, offering support for a variety of daily tasks [7]. OrCam's devices are distributed across several countries and available in over 25 languages, allowing it to reach a significant international user base, especially among the estimated 300 million people worldwide who live with visual impairment. In Romania, this device is provided free to individuals with a handicap certificate, aged 18 to 65. Since the initiative began, it has aimed to support about 7000 people, although the exact number of current users remains unspecified. The company offers full support in Romania, assisting with application processes and visiting patients multiple times to set up and adjust the device. These technologies significantly improve independence by providing audible access to visual information, including texts, faces, products, and colors.

NuEyes is a technology company specializing in wearable, hands-free devices designed to enhance vision for individuals with low vision or blindness. Their products, such as electronic smart glasses, use advanced augmented reality (AR) and virtual reality (VR) technologies to magnify and clarify objects in the user's environment, making daily tasks like reading, watching TV, or recognizing faces much easier. The lightweight and comfortable designs allow users to maintain a natural head posture, making them suitable for extended use. With voice-controlled features, NuEyes glasses provide accessibility without requiring complex hand movements, which is particularly beneficial for users with limited dexterity. Through these innovations, NuEyes aims to improve quality of life and promote independence for people experiencing vision loss due to conditions such as macular degeneration, glaucoma, and diabetic retinopathy [8].

eSight 3 and eSight 4 are innovative electronic eyewear designed to assist individuals with low vision, offering advanced technology to enhance their visual experience. The eSight 3 model features high-definition cameras and sophisticated image processing algorithms that capture real-time video and display it on two screens, allowing users to see their environment more clearly. It is lightweight and adjustable, making it comfortable for extended wear. The eSight 4 model builds on this foundation with improved image quality, a more streamlined design, and enhanced features such as a larger field of view and customizable settings to adapt to different lighting conditions. Both versions empower users to engage in daily activities, such as reading, watching TV, and navigating their surroundings, promoting greater independence and a better quality of life for those with visual impairments [9].

Modern canes for visually impaired individuals are equipped with advanced technologies, such as ultrasonic sensors and GPS, to enhance navigation and obstacle detection. These smart canes provide real-time feedback through vibrations or audio cues, helping users to safely navigate their environments while promoting greater independence. Cane FB Reader is an innovative device designed to assist individuals who are visually impaired or blind by enabling them to access printed text independently. This portable reader utilizes advanced optical character recognition (OCR) technology to scan text from books, documents, and other printed materials, converting it into clear audio output. Compact and user-friendly, the Cane FB Reader is easy to carry and operate, making it ideal for daily use at home, school, work, or while traveling. The device also includes adjustable speech settings, allowing users to customize reading speed and voice type according to their preferences. By bridging the gap between printed text and audio, the Cane FB Reader helps promote greater independence and accessibility for those with visual impairments, enhancing both learning opportunities and quality of life [10]. The AMAIS ultrasound cane is an assistive device for visually impaired individuals that incorporates ultrasonic sensors to detect obstacles. By emitting ultrasonic waves, the cane identifies objects at various distances, alerting the user through tactile or auditory feedback to ensure safer navigation in unfamiliar or complex environments. This technology enhances traditional cane functionality, providing more proactive obstacle avoidance for users [11].

A novel system was designed to help visually impaired individuals navigate indoor environments independently [12]. This system uses a hybrid infrastructure of RFID and Bluetooth Low Energy (BLE) to provide location and orientation information. By creating a chain of destination points based on the user's input, the system enables users to navigate complex spaces by optimizing paths through an algorithm similar to the traveling salesman problem. Designed with a user-friendly interface, the system gives real-time guidance, making navigation more efficient and secure. Tested in a hospital setting, the system proved effective in aiding visually impaired individuals, who were able to reach specific locations through voice-guided instructions delivered via a smartphone. This technology is intended for environments with complex layouts, like hospitals or large public buildings, and has shown promising results in preliminary trial [12].

In today's technologically advanced world, numerous applications are designed to empower individuals with visual impairments, enhancing their independence and quality of life. These innovative apps harness the power of artificial intelligence, augmented reality, and optical character recognition to provide users with tools that facilitate navigation, reading, and everyday tasks. From smartphone apps that describe the environment and read text aloud to wearable devices that detect obstacles, these solutions help bridge the gap between visual limitations and the ability to interact with the world. By leveraging the capabilities of modern technology, these applications support individuals and promote inclusivity and accessibility, ensuring that people with vision impairments can engage more fully with their surroundings.

Digit-Eyes is an app designed to help visually impaired individuals identify products and organize items independently. By scanning barcodes on products, Digit-Eyes provides audio descriptions, including item names, ingredients, and handling instructions. Additionally, it allows users to create custom, scannable labels for personal belongings, enabling easy identification of items at home or in storage. Users can print labels using any standard printer, making the app versatile and adaptable for a variety of organizational needs. With its accessible design, Digit-Eyes empowers users to confidently manage daily tasks, enhancing their autonomy and quality of life [13]. Envision AI is a powerful app that leverages artificial intelligence to assist visually impaired individuals in perceiving and understanding their surroundings. Using the smartphone camera, Envision AI can recognize text, objects, colors, and even people, delivering spoken descriptions to the user. The app reads documents, labels, and signs aloud and can process handwritten text, making it a versatile tool for reading in diverse settings. Envision AI also supports facial recognition, allowing users to identify familiar faces in real time, and offers currency and color recognition for everyday tasks. Through intuitive design and advanced AI, Envision AI empowers users to navigate daily life with greater independence and confidence [14].

Seeing AI is a groundbreaking app developed by Microsoft designed to assist individuals with visual impairments by converting the visual world into an audible experience. Using the camera on a smartphone, Seeing AI can recognize and describe various elements, including people, text, objects, and even currency, providing real-time audio feedback to users. It features multiple modes, such as reading printed text aloud, identifying products through barcode scanning, and recognizing the emotions of people in the vicinity, enhancing social interactions. The app's user-friendly interface allows users to customize settings to suit their needs, making it a versatile tool for navigating everyday situations. By transforming how visually impaired individuals interact with their surroundings, Seeing AI promotes greater independence and enriches daily experiences, empowering users to engage more fully with the world around them [15]. Supersense is an innovative app designed to assist visually impaired individuals by using artificial intelligence to interpret the surrounding environment through a smartphone's camera. The app provides real-time audio descriptions of objects, people, and text, helping users navigate their surroundings with greater confidence and independence. With features like barcode scanning, currency recognition, and a simple user interface, Supersense enhances everyday activities and fosters a more inclusive experience for its users [16].

Conclusion

Adapting computer programs to support visually impaired individuals is not just a matter of accessibility; it is a crucial step towards fostering inclusivity and independence in our increasingly digital world. By leveraging technologies such as screen readers, voice recognition, and adaptive interfaces, developers can create software that empowers users to engage with information and tools that many take for granted. As society continues to embrace innovation, it is essential to prioritize the needs of individuals with special needs, in the design and the implementation of the computer programs. Through collaboration and a commitment to accessibility, we can ensure that technology serves as a bridge, rather than a barrier, enabling everyone to participate fully in the digital age.

Disclaimer

This paper was first presented at the CONFERENCE Family medicine, the cornerstone of modern medicine, 15th Edition

Volume of summaries, September 5-7, 2024, Etna medical publishing house, ISBN 978-630-6644-03-2.

References

[1] Ioana Soare. Criterii de pensionare în oftalmologie. Viața medicală; 2019.

[2] Legea nr. 448/2006 privind protecţia și promovarea drepturilor persoanelor cu handicap,

http://www.mmuncii.ro/pub/imagemanager/images/file/Legislatie/LEGI/L448-2006_rep.pdf.
[3] Ioana Soare. Expertiză medicală. Medicină de asigurări. Editura Etna; 2017.
[4] Anthony Candela. Legends and Pioneers of Blindness Assistive Technology, Part 3. American Foundation for the Blind https://www.afb.org/aw/7/6/14413.
[5] Jiménez J, Olea J, Torres J, Alonso I, Harder D, Fischer K. Biography of Louis Braille and invention of the Braille alphabet. Surv Ophthalmol. 2009;54(1):142-149. doi:10.1016/j.survophthal.2008.10.006.
[6] Jiaji Wang, Shuihua Wang, Yudong Zhang. Artificial intelligence for visually impaired. Displays. Volume 77; 2023 https://doi.org/10.1016/j.displa.2023.102391.
[7] Nguyen XT, Koopman J, van Genderen MM, Stam HLM, Boon CJF. Artificial vision: the effectiveness of the OrCam in patients with advanced inherited retinal dystrophies. Acta Ophthalmol. 2022 Jun;100(4):e986-e993. doi: 10.1111/aos.15001.
[8] https://www.nueyes.com/
[9] https://www.esighteyewear.com/
[10] Hersh M. Wearable Travel Aids for Blind and Partially Sighted People: A Review with a Focus on Design Issues. Sensors (Basel). 2022; 22(14):5454. doi:10.3390/s22145454
[11] https://en.ceciaa.com/ultracane.html
[12] Kahraman, M., & Turhan, C. (2021). An intelligent indoor guidance and navigation system for the visually impaired. Assistive Technology, 34(4), 478–486. https://doi.org/10.1080/10400435.2021.1872738
[13] https://www.digit-eyes.com/
[14] https://www.letsenvision.com/
[15] https://www.perkins.org/resource/seeing-ai-ios-app-recognizing-people-objects-and-scenes/
[16] https://www.supersense.app/product-page-supersense

PART 8

RELATION WITH OCCUPATIONAL MEDICINE

CHAPTER 1

WORK ACCIDENTS

IOANA SOARE AND ANCA PAVEL

The work accident is represented by the violent injury to the body, as well as the acute professional intoxication, which occur during the work process or in the performance of work duties and which cause temporary incapacity for work for at least 3 days, disability or death [1].

It may be called workplace injury, workplace accident, industrial accident, industry injury, occupational injury.

The work accident is not an inevitable phenomenon, it can be prevented and combated if all hygiene and work protection measures are taken and respected.

In order to be taken into account as a work accident, the existence of an employment contract between the employer and the employee is necessary [2]. The following are also considered work accidents:

- Accidents suffered by pupils, students, apprentices, the unemployed, during professional practice and by staff working during the trial period or during professional courses.
- Accident suffered by persons performing state or public interest tasks;
- Accident that occurred during cultural and sports activities organized by authorized institutions
- Accident suffered by any person, as a result of an action taken on their own initiative to save human lives or to prevent or eliminate a danger that threatens public property;
- Road accident, if the journey to work was made during and on a normal route;
- Accident during the journey from one office or place of work to another

- Accident suffered in the performance of work duties, as a result of an assault
- Accident caused by natural phenomena or calamities, if the victim was fulfilling his duties
- Disappearance of a person in the conditions of a work accident and in circumstances that justify the assumption of his death [1].

The following generally are **not considered work accidents:**

- Accidents caused by external, major events not related to work (e.g. terrorist attacks or natural disasters).
- Accidents caused by the recklessness of a worker.
- Accidents caused by another worker that are not related to work (e.g. fights or pranks between workers that result in injury).
- Accidents suffered as a result of intentional crimes being committed [3].

Work accidents are classified into:

- Accident causing temporary incapacity for work
- Accident causing disability
- Accident causing death
- Collective accident [1].

THE PATIENT PATH is currently carried out according to law 360/2023, the law on pensions and other social security rights, law 346/2002 and the law on safety and health at work, 319/2006, in Romania.

Any event or accident, possibly a work accident, will be communicated to the management of the respective company. A representative of it has the obligation to communicate the event within 48 hours from the date of production, to the local Labor Protection Inspectorate (Romania) [1]. Then an investigation commission is chosen and the FIAM, the work accident registration form, is filled out.

In the event of a work accident, after providing first aid at the workplace or at the hospital, possibly hospitalization, the medical certificate of temporary incapacity for work is issued, which will bear the mention EMERGENCY and will not be coded for work accidents, because the research was not yet done. After obtaining FIAM, form of registered work accident, the medical certificates will be able to be coded work accident.

Groups sensitive to specific risks, such as: pregnant or nursing women, the elderly, young people, as well as people with disabilities, must be protected against the dangers that affect them specifically and the workplace must be adapted.

The consequences of work accidents, resulting in the loss of a certain percentage of work capacity, will be medically evaluated. This percentage must be determined by the insurance doctors of the National House of Public Pensions (CNPP).

The claim for compensation will bring the patient the financial compensation provided by law, i.e., as the case may be, disability pension or compensatory payments from the National House of Public Pensions.

The insured have the right to medical benefits for the rehabilitation of health and the recovery of work capacity [1].

In Romania, the recovery treatments provided for in art. 23 paragraph (1) c), d) and e) from Law no. 346/2002, necessary after the discharge of the insured, must be analyzed and approved by their social insurance expert doctor from the medical expertise service within the territorial pension houses.

(2) Tickets for spa treatment, provided in art. 25 para. (3) from Law no. 346/2002, will be granted in accordance with the criteria established by decision of the NHPP president.

Reparative surgery is intended only for cases involving the restoration of work capacity, the loss of which resulted from a work accident or a confirmed occupational disease.

ART. 22

(1) The insured benefits, upon request, from the granting of aid for the procurement of medical devices in order to correct and recover organic, functional or physical deficiencies in cases of work accidents or occupational diseases, according to the provisions of art. 24 para. (1) from Law no. 346/2002.

The insured have the right to benefits and services regarding professional rehabilitation and reconversion, in accordance with the provisions of Law 346/2002.

Compensation for temporary work incapacity/short term sick leave/medical leave is granted for a maximum of 183 days in a year, counted from the first day of illness, in Romania. Starting with the 90th day, the medical leave can be extended up to 183 days, with the approval of the social insurance medical expert [4]. The extension of medical leave, beyond 183 days, is done for a maximum of 90 days, according to the procedures established by the NHPP, in relation to the evolution of the case and the results of recovery actions.

The patient has the right to allowance for temporary transfer to another job and allowance for reducing working time by 25%, which is granted on the medical leave certificate, for 90 days per year.

Compensation for achieving integrity

The insured have the right to compensations for achieving integrity, in accordance with the provisions of Law 346/2002.

Compensation in the event of death is a fixed amount, it is granted from the Work Accident Fund based on the application submitted to the Department of Work Accidents in the public pension houses, in Romania.

Cases discussed

- **problems in France** - 56 years old man, working in the night shift as manufacturing operator in an industrial pastry company, suffered a myocardial infarction, declared work accident (in Romania we do not declare myocardial infarction as work accident). Occupational exposure: handling weights, repetitive movements, prolonged standing, flour powder, postural stress on the spine. He was evaluated at occupational medicine in the pre-half visit (during medical leave), in order to assess the possibility of resuming professional activity. The pre-work sheet was made with recommendations for arranging the workplace or reclassification to an administrative, sedentary position, respecting the contraindications for carrying weights, night work, with the possibility to sit down if necessary. It was recommended to temporarily reduce the working time to 50%, maximum 4 hours per day, possibility existing after WA for one year, with salary compensation by social insurance. Any arrangement of the workplace required the employer's consent, which was obtained but for another job, order preparation.

He took a procedure called "framed test". The procedure involves an attempt to resume the activity, for a defined period of time, under the observation of a guardian appointed by the employer, who makes a written report sent to the partners who have previously approved the procedure: the occupational physician, the family physician, the social security consultant physician, the employer and coordinator of the PDP cell (prevention in professional disintegration).

For this patient, the observation lasted a week (5 days), the report being favorable. The result of the report allowed the delivery of a fitness certificate (Fit for Work) by the occupational physician, during the half-time visit, for the post arranged at 1/2 the norm, in compliance with the contraindications listed in the pre-half time sheet.

He resumed activity, as a protected employee.

The enterprise was sold. The owner change meant also the change of organization. The new employer refused the continuation of the part-time activity, imposed the resumption of the full-time activity or the reassessment of the aptitude. The employee did not accept the idea of a professional reconversion, necessarily wanting to work full time. Gradually, the boss no longer respected any medical contraindications, which led to a conflict between the two.

The current situation, after full-time activity, without medical leave, with WA consolidated with 5% sequelae, with a quasi-normal cardio consultation, did not allow either unfitness or referral to the consulting doctor for a possible disability (for chronic coronary disease, unrelated with WA).

Therefore, the 3 options were taken into account:

- Continuation of the activity, without setting up the post
- Conventional break, with unemployment benefit for 2 years maximum
- Resignation, no right to unemployment.

The patient was no longer followed by the occupational physician.

- problems in Romania [4]

1. An 18-year-old boy, suffered an accident at work with the amputation of his right hand, two days after employment, on a modified machine (the manual lever was adapted for the foot - so that the worker had free hands!!!).

Admitted to the hospital, he was denied the right to medical leave, because he did not have the necessary contribution period, and the work accident was not declared. The patient was still paid his salary at work, but after two months he was informed that he had to solve his situation, which is why he presented himself at the medical expertise office. He was advised to report the accident to the Bucharest Labor Inspectorate. After 2 months, he received at home a report for work accident. Since the company refused to pay him medical leave or to change his job, the patient has received disability pension (2004). We mention that he was a young patient, able to perform another activity after receiving a prosthetic hand and retrained.

2. Patient with undeclared work accident, with cranio-cervical trauma, multiple wounds and damage to the nerves of the left upper limb, presented for disability retirement in March 2005. In the file there were two hospital discharge letters, as well as a statement of the guard who found the casualty. The statement of findings has not been completed. The patient came to work on a Saturday, at his normal workplace but not in the normal program. The patient was referred to the Bucharest Labor Inspectorate, with the closing of the file postponed until the cause of the disability was clarified. The work accident was declared.

3. Patient with calf fracture due to road accident, declared that he had the accident during working hours, when he went out with his colleagues - he jumped the fence - to drink a beer at the bar across the street. The company refused to declare WA.

4. Patient with an accident at work, outside of working hours - he had come to process a piece for himself and cut several of his fingers. The company refused to issue an WA report.

5. Patient with a fall accident, calf fracture, during office hours, at a client's office, where he had gone to fill out some documents, being sent by the employer. After recovery, he is reinstated at work. A year later, in the same place and conditions, he suffered a second accident with a calf fracture in the same leg. This time too, WA was not declared. The 38-year-old patient received disability pension.

6. Alcoholic patient, with personality disorders, civilian employee at a military unit, slips and spills a basin of sulfuric acid on his pants. He was not wearing a protective uniform. He suffered a II-III degree burn on his right lower limb. The unit refused to declare WA. The unit doctor had

declared him unfit for work, but they had no way to move him to another job or a legal basis to fire him. The patient received disability pension.

7. The patient, a maid at a student dormitory, slipped on the stairs at work and suffered a calf fracture. No WA was declared. The patient received disability pension, as for a common disease.

- international problems - Work Accidents Abroad

1997 - 35 Romanian opera singers were involved in a bus accident in Germany, with 4 of them ending up hospitalised there, then sent home.

2005-2007 -While on a cruise, 3 waiters and a singer slipped and fell. They were hospitalised, then sent home.

2009 - A captain returning home from the ship had a car accident, with multiple fractures and organ lesions.

1998-2002 - 3 constructions workers in Israel fell from a building, were hospitalised, then sent home.

2010 - A professional soldier, hurt by a blast in Afghanistan, was hospitalised, then sent home.

THESE WORK ACCIDENTS WERE NEVER DECLARED.

After being injured, the workers were sent to their own country to be evaluated by the insurance doctor. The diagnosis report was then sent to the insurance company, whether local or foreign, which was then interpreted according to different translations of the same terms.

It is most often that money, insurance funds, are paid by the native country in most cases. Only when the patient was life insured, he received money from the private insurer. The laws still differ from country to country, and so do the forms. The EU standard forms are still generally unknown to the medical community.

References

1. Law 319/2006, safety and health at work, https://www.inspectiamuncii.ro/documents/66402/267247/Legea+319+din+2006.pdf/20e92134-6870-4776-9417-840a89a852b3
2. Law 346/2002, regarding insurance for work accidents and occupational diseases, https://legislatie.just.ro/Public/DetaliiDocument/36905 - law 346/2002
3. https://www.topdoctors.co.uk/medical-dictionary/work-accidents
4. Soare Ioana, Medical Expertise, Insurance Medicine, Editura Etna, Bucuresti, 2017

CHAPTER 2

OCCUPATIONAL DISEASES

IOANA SOARE, ANCA PAVEL
AND VALENTIN EUGEN CIOCSAN

It is also called occupational illness, work illness, industrial illness, industrial disease, industrial disorder, professional disease.

An **'occupational disease'** is any disease caused primarily by exposure at work to a physical, organizational, chemical or biological risk factor or to a combination of these factors. Occupational diseases are mostly those listed in national legislation as resulting from exposure to risk factors at work. The recognition of an occupational disease may be linked to a compensation, if it is clear that there is a causal relationship between an occupational exposure and the disease [1].

Occupational diseases occur as a result of exercising a job or profession, caused by harmful factors, as well as by overstraining the body during the work process [2].

The Canadian Centre for Occupational Health and Safety (CCOHS) states that "In general, health conditions or disorders that occur among a group of people with similar occupational exposures at a higher frequency than the rest of the population are considered to be occupational diseases."

There is a separate category, diseases related to the profession, with multifactorial etiology, in which some determining factors are of a professional nature. A **'work-related disease'** is any illness caused or made worse by workplace factors. This includes many diseases that have more complex causes, involving a combination of occupational and non-work-related factors [1]. The Canadian Centre for Occupational Health and Safety (CCOHS) states that "In general, health conditions or disorders that occur among a group of people with similar occupational exposures at a higher frequency than the rest of the population are considered to be occupational diseases."

Work-related diseases include:

- Musculoskeletal disorders
- Stress and mental health disorders
- Work-related cancer
- Skin diseases
- Work-related diseases from biological agents [1].

There are two special cases:

- Acute occupational poisoning is also declared as work accident
- Occupational communicable disease is also declared a communicable disease (ex. COVID for medical staff) [2].

In order to be taken into account as an occupational disease, the existence of an employment contract between the employer and the employee is necessary. Also considered occupational diseases in Romania, are the ailments produced under the conditions stated above, ailments suffered by pupils, students, apprentices, during professional practice and by staff working during the trial period [2].

The list of occupational diseases whose declaration, research and records are mandatory in Romania are presented in HG 1425/ 2006, Annex 22 [3].

International Labour Organization has a List of Occupational Diseases, as the least recommended to be declared. Each country has its own list of occupational diseases, some being locally specific.

The consequences of occupational diseases, resulting in the loss of a certain percentage of work capacity, must be medically evaluated. This percentage must be determined by the insurance doctors of the National House of Pension and Other Rights of Social Insurance (CNPP), in Romania.

The claim will bring the patient the financial compensation provided by law, i.e., as the case may be, disability pension degree I, II or III or compensatory payments from the CNPP.

The insured have the right to medical benefits for the rehabilitation of health and the recovery of work capacity, in accordance with the provisions of Law

346/2002 on insurance for occupational accidents and occupational diseases and the methodological norms approved by Order no. 450/825.

The recovery treatments provided for in art. 23 para. (1) lit. c), d) and e) from Law no. 346/2002, necessary after the discharge of the insured, must be analyzed and approved by their social insurance expert doctor from the medical expertise service within the territorial pension houses.

In Great Britain Regulation 8 of the Reporting of Injuries, Diseases and Dangerous Occurrences Regulations (RIDDOR) requires employers and self-employed people to report cases of certain diagnosed reportable diseases. These must be linked to exposure to specified hazards at work [4]. Only a few conditions are mentioned:

- Carpal tunnel syndrome
- Hand or forearm cramps
- Occupational dermatitis
- Hand-arm vibration syndrome
- Occupational asthma
- Tendinitis or tenosynovitis [4].

There is guidance on carcinogens, mutagens and biological agents that explains when employers and self-employed workers must report:

- any disease caused by an occupational exposure to a biological agent,
- cases of occupational cancer [4].

The employer's measures to prevent the occurrence of these diseases are considered. And hence the problem of another section of the DWP, guided by the written and detailed conclusions of the medical assessor.

Form DA1 (formerly E123) is the Certificate of entitlement to medical treatment under special conditions reserved for accidents at work and occupational diseases in another EU country [5].

Occupational disease is not an inevitable phenomenon, it can be prevented and fought if all hygiene and work protection measures are taken and respected.

References

1. https://osha.europa.eu/en/themes/work-related-diseases
2. https://legislatie.just.ro/Public/DetaliiDocument/36905 - law 346/2002, regarding insurance for work accidents and occupational diseases
3. https://www.iprotectiamuncii.ro/legi/hg-1425-2006.pdf
4. https://www.hse.gov.uk/riddor/occupational-diseases.htm
5. https://europa.eu/youreurope/citizens/work/social-security-and-benefits/social-security-forms/index_en.htm, visited 14.12.2024

PART 9

ETHICS

CHAPTER 1

PROFESSIONAL ETHICS OF THE INSURANCE PHYSICIAN

ROXANA MIRICA AND IOANA SOARE

The medical profession is based on ethical statements [1], commitments, responsibilities and the highest standards, which guide physicians in fulfilling their obligation to provide [2] competent medical care [1] for the patients. The oldest mentions are in the Hammurabi code and the most used ethical code for doctors is The Hippocratic Oath.

The World Medical Association (WMA) has developed the International Code of Medical Ethics as an ethical principle for the medical profession worldwide [3]. According to Declaration of Geneva of 1975 "The Physician's Pledge and the WMA's entire body of policies, define and elucidate the professional duties of physicians towards their patients, other physicians and health professionals, themselves and society as a whole." [3]

In Romania, the control of the practice of the medical profession is carried out by the Romanian College of Physicians and the Ministry of Health [4,5].

The Social Health Insurance System (Bismarck type) is based on compulsory societal contributions related to the income, protecting the whole population of the country such as wage earners, the pensioners, even the unemployed. having the obligation to assure their health according to the law [6].

The national code of medical ethics governs the work of every physician. Due to the particular content, scope, and setting of insurance medicine, supplementary guidelines of conduct are needed [7].

Professional ethics constitute a necessity, so that the activity of the social insurance physicians can enjoy credibility, acceptance and a good reputation [7], establishing its code on a series of fundamental principles:

1. The primary duty of the physician is to promote the health and well-being of the patients [4].
2. The physician must practice medicine fairly, justly [4], competently [3], with conscience, honesty, compassion, humility and prudence [3] – **professional integrity**
3. The physician must provide health care based on patient's needs without bias or discrimination [3], respecting the dignity, autonomy and rights of the claimant and other parties involved and treats them empathetically [7] – **professional objectivity**
4. The doctors must avoid real or potential conflicts of interest in a professional manner while exercising **independent professional judgement** [3]. Independence represents the main means by which the social insurance physicians demonstrates that they can fulfill their mission objectively, it ensures principlism and verticality in respecting the law, the correctness of the reports, the consistency and firmness of the professional in promoting deontology [6] and recognizing a responsibility to seek changes in those requirements which are contrary to the best interests of the patient [2].
5. The physician must be familiarized with the health condition of the claimant based on all the information provided, clarifying the intention of medical actions such as physical examination of the claimant and consideration of the claimant's self-report, informing the claimant about every phase of the care process and the procedure of the insurance medical assessment [7] and respecting the patient's decision to withhold or withdraw consent for any reason [4].
6. The **professional secrecy** represents the patient's privacy and maintain the confidentiality consistent with the code of medical ethics and applicable regulations [7], with the exception of situations in which it is expressly authorized for this purpose or there are legal provisions for disclosure such as the case of criminal acts [6].
7. The doctors must establish appropriate insurance physicians-claimant relationship [7], through professional boundaries [4].
8. The physician must not allow to be influenced by possibility of accepting benefits/fees for services for themselves or for the institution, dependent upon writing a report, favorable to any party [7].
9. Understanding objectively and independently all the statues and laws regulations that form the basis for insurance and health related benefits [7].
10. The conclusions of the social insurance assessment must provide a proper medical justification based on high professional standards, a

solid medical knowledge and adequate qualifications of the independent medical evaluator [7].

11. A physician should participate in medical activities [4], maintain a commitment to medical education, share scientific knowledge [2] and expertise for the benefit of patients [4], contributing to the improvement of the betterment of public and global health [2].
12. The physician must engage with other health professionals in a respectful and collaborative manner, ensuring that ethical principles are upheld when working in teams [4].
13. In the relationship with the society, the doctors must recognize that social determinants of health, the environment and other fundamental factors are important items that affect the health of the patient and of the population [3].

Conclusions

Insurance medical experts are included in a larger family of judicial and extrajudicial experts.

Accountants, technical experts (in constructions or most known, in car damage) all have a conduct code [8,].

Independence as a principle - all those ethical codes for “other” experts differentiate between “hired professional” and “professional in public practice” [10,11].

Is it ethical to hire an insurance medical expert in an insurance company? Can or may hired physicians represent the best interesses of the patient?

Should the medical expert be independent?

References

1. AMA Principles of Medical Ethics. Adopted June 1957; revised June 1980; revised June 2001. https://code-medical-ethics.ama-assn.org/principles
2. Canadian Medical Association Code of Ethics and Professionalism; December 2018 https://www.cma.ca/cma-code-ethics-and-professionalism
3. World Medical Association International Code of Medical Ethics, October 2022. https://www.wma.net/policies-post/wma-international-code-of-medical-ethics/

4. The Code of Medical Ethics of the Romanian College of Physicians. Law 306/ 2004.
5. Law 95/2006, on health care reform, https://legislatie.just.ro/Public/DetaliiDocument/71139
6. Văidean Viorela-Ligia, Nistor Ioan, The social health insurances in Romania – realities and perspectives, 2010; https://doctorat.ubbcluj.ro/sustinerea_publica/rezumate/2010/finante/Vaidean_Viorela_EN.pdf
7. Guidelines of Conduct for Insurance Physicians – European Union of Medicine in Assurance and Social Security https://eumass.eu/guidelines-of-conduct-for-insurance-physicians-3/
8. Boulescu Mircea, Ghita Marcel. Accounting expertise, Didactic and Pedagogical Publishing House, 2001
9. AGIR, AEXEA, SETEC, Independent extrajudicial technical expert and consultant, AGIR Publishing House, 2010
10. https://ceccar.ro/ro/wp-content/uploads/2011/09/Codul_etic_2011.pdf
11. https://www.icaew.com/-/media/corporate/files/members/regulations-standards-and-guidance/ethics/icaew-code-of-ethics-2020.ashx#page=3
12. https://inml-mm.ro/doc/pdf/cod-etica-medic-legist.pdf
13. ACFEI American College of Forensic Examiners International Archived 7/25/2005
14. Experts – overriding duty to the court Civil English law (Instruction of Experts to give Evidence in Civil Claims)
15. Canadian Society of Forensic Science, Rules of Professional Conduct, adopted November 5, 1994
16. Australian and New Zealand Forensic Science Society Archived 7/25/2005

CHAPTER 2

DISCRIMINATION IN INSURANCE MEDICINE

IOANA SOARE

United States

Under the Affordable Care Act, since 2014, the insurance companies were no longer allowed to deny coverage or impose limitations based on the pre-existing conditions.

Americans with Disabilities Act (ADA),3 Section 504 of the Rehabilitation Act of 1973 (Section 504),4 and Section 1557 of the Patient Protection and Affordable Care Act (Section 1557).5 Each of these federal laws protects people with disabilities from discrimination based on their disability. Section 504 is the part of the Rehabilitation Act that prohibits discrimination [1].

The US Rehabilitation Act of 1973 and the Americans with Disabilities Act (ADA), since 1992, prohibits from discriminating against qualified individuals with disabilities in job application procedures, hiring, firing, advancement, compensation, job training, or in the terms, conditions and privileges of employment. Companies must make "reasonable accommodation" to people with different needs. Protection is extended to anyone with (A) a physical or mental impairment that substantially limits one or more of the major life activities of an individual, (B) a record of such an impairment, or (C) being regarded as having such an impairment. The second and third criteria are seen as ensuring protection from unjust discrimination based on a perception of risk, just because someone has a record of impairment or appears to have a disability or illness (e.g. features which may be erroneously taken as signs of an illness) [1].

United Kingdom

Under the Disability Discrimination Act (DDA) (1995, extended in 2005), it is unlawful for the organizations to discriminate (treat a disabled person less favorably, for reasons related to the person's disability, without justification) in the employment; access to goods, facilities, services; managing, buying or renting land or property; education. Businesses must make "reasonable adjustments" to their policies or practices, or physical aspects of their premises, to avoid indirect discrimination [2].

Discrimination in employment

A number of financial and care support services are available, including Incapacity Benefit and Disability Living Allowance.

African Americans and disability

According to the 2000 U.S. Census, the African American community has the highest rate of disability at 20.8 percent, slightly higher than the overall disability rate of 19.4%. There still remains a stigma attached to the disability.

African Americans with a disability are subject to not only this stigma but also to the race discrimination. Doctor Eddie Glenn of Howard University describes this situation as the "triple jeopardy" syndrome: African American women who have a disability face tremendous discrimination due to their condition, race, and gender [2].

Disability rights movement

The disability rights movement, led by the individuals with disabilities, began in the 1970s. This self-advocacy is often seen as largely responsible for the shift toward independent living and accessibility. The term "Independent Living" was taken from 1959 California legislation which enabled people who had acquired a disability due to polio to leave hospital wards and move back into the community with the help of cash benefits for the purchase of personal assistance with the activities of daily living.

With its origins in the U.S. civil rights and the consumer movements of the late 1960s, the movement and its philosophy have since spread to other continents influencing self-perception, organization and social policy [2,3].

Conclusions

Maybe someday we will all talk the same "language", we will all understand what we are talking about – insurance/ assurance – pension/benefit/allowance.

We all work to help our employers to save money in insurance businesses. For the sake of the psychological approach the Britons have used in the last 10 years, we all should no longer use words as benefit, allowance, handicap, invalid, pension.

So, let's go down to basics and call all these money for short-term sick leave, money for long-term sick leave (or money for health care, more difficult to spend on alcohol and cigarettes), not pension – which is for life, earned by yourself, not allowance – which is something you are allowed to have, benefit – which is something you receive as a bonus, premium, from bene – good, facere – to do – something you receive from the will of somebody to do some good.

Politically correct is not "handicapped" persons, not even persons with handicap, not invalid persons – meaning not valid/ not normal, not a whole. Correct would be to call them persons with disabilities or persons with special needs.

References

1. https://www.hhs.gov/sites/default/files/ocr/civilrights/resources/factsheets/504.pdf
2. Shakespeare Tom, Disability, The Basics, Routledge, 2018, p 1-5, p 56
3. www.aaimedicine.org

CHAPTER 3

DISCRIMINATION FACED BY WHEELCHAIR USERS IN HEALTHCARE

STEFAN MOSHE STOIAN

As a legal expert and an individual with mobility challenges, I have taken on the role of an independent specialist for the Monitoring Council overseeing the enforcement of the Convention on the Rights of Persons with Disabilities. This convention was adopted by the United Nations General Assembly in New York on December 13, 2006, signed by Romania on September 26, 2007, and ratified by Romania through Law 221/2010.

The absence of a point of contact within the Romanian Ministry of Transport for users of technology in travel, mobility, and transport creates significant challenges. To ensure timely access, we have created the Facebook page "Coalitia nedeplasabilului" https://www.facebook.com/groups/779799468763551 for individuals with similar disabilities, aiming to find a as uniform a solution as possible. It is essential that whenever we address discrimination, we clarify whether it is viewed negatively or positively, along with the criteria on which the principle of equal opportunities will be applied to realize the asserted right.

The fundamental principle of applying non-discrimination seeks to create equal opportunities for all citizens in relation to each of the fundamental rights outlined in international, community, and national law. Consequently, every citizen should have equal access to rights such as education, training, health care, culture, transportation, housing, property, income, and mobility, among others. The methods through which states are required to guarantee this equal access can vary in nature or be of similar types, but differ in their intensity. Therefore, to address negative discrimination that is prohibited, states must assess, justify, and propose specific measures for each distinct criterion of discrimination.

For these reasons, the legal framework differentiates between discrimination, non-discrimination, and anti-discrimination.

Positive anti-discrimination initiatives promote non-discrimination and are encouraged by secondary legislation, while they are mandatory under primary legislation, particularly in relation to Article 14 of the ECHR and the Romanian Constitution, which asserts in Article 16 that negative discrimination is not allowed.

My expertise pertains to the non-discrimination of real estate; specifically, I am qualified to identify, implement, and advocate for precise measures to address unfair treatment in order to provide equal opportunities for individuals whose mobility relies on assistive technologies, access infrastructure, transportation, lifting methods, or similar means for entering buildings. We are also addressing the structures that are inaccessible to individuals with all types of mobility impairments.

To utilize these services, the physical environment's accessibility, the communication environment, and the entitlement to health, recovery, and medical rehabilitation must be confirmed. Concerning access to the physical environment, it should be designed to accommodate individuals with special needs in all buildings and throughout all pathways, streets, or corridors from their home to the medical service provider's location. Any service provider lacking complete accessibility in their infrastructure should have their operating license revoked, along with their right to practice.

The liability insurance of a clinic authorized to operate in an inaccessible building should include insurance premiums, that guarantee adequate compensation for individuals with medical recommendations or referrals who are unable to access medical services, due to physical barriers.

Additionally, access to petitioning is also restricted.

Regarding physical accessibility, mobile elevators cannot be refused, based on the argument that they might be operated by the owner's employees outside their working hours or during the personal rehabilitation and social integration programs of individuals with disabilities who rely on personal assistance.

Furthermore, some individuals with disabilities may not have an official disability certificate or may be in a temporary or undiagnosed motor disability situation. However, they still have the right to access services in some inaccessible environments.

Israeli law permits the demolition of unlawfully constructed discriminatory infrastructure and could serve as a model of best practices.

To enhance accessibility, it is essential to establish a dedicated contact point in each city for individuals with reduced mobility seeking medical tourism. This would facilitate technologically assisted travel with professionally trained assistants, to ensure safety.

Additionally, the creation of an international short-number helpline would be beneficial, allowing individuals to request mobility technologies and live assistance to navigate infrastructure more effectively.

Regarding communication access, all medical service providers should be required to publish their work schedules online, provide a registration number upon written patient requests, and ensure document submission to specialists. They should also maintain WhatsApp communication with individuals reliant on mobility technologies, ensuring continuous accessibility in consideration of their needs.

In the family medicine, bedridden or immobile patients should receive prescription medications online, directly accessible at nearby pharmacies, while referral tickets should be delivered via courier.

Moreover, a referral ticket should be required for transport using emergency non-medically assisted ambulances. To facilitate independent transportation for individuals dependent on mobility technologies to outpatient clinics or medical service providers, specialized vehicles must be made available.

The quality of accessibility in buildings and transportation infrastructure is primarily determined by those who rely on the mobility technologies, and it should not be assessed by individuals who do not use such aids. Additionally, every disability is unique, requiring personalized solutions. Mobility technologies serve as essential tools, that enhance each individual's ability to move independently to the greatest extent possible.

The physical environment must be designed to accommodate the safe and effective use of these technologies and devices.

In Romania, significant improvements are needed in the quality of family medicine services, particularly in cases where they are provided in ground-floor apartments that are incompatible with mobility technologies or lack safe accessibility.

The state has a responsibility to establish accessibility standards, ensuring the construction of concrete or asphalt ramps, that provide adequate traction for wheelchair rubber wheels. No ground floor should lack a ramp, and no upper floor should be without an elevator.

While inaccessibility should be the exception, it remains the norm, as the built environment and infrastructure frequently fail to accommodate all individuals and the mobility technologies they rely on for free movement.

Liability insurance for family medicine services should cover far more than current provisions, especially for individuals with severe mobility limitations.

Furthermore, it is essential to recognize that immobile patients require all medical consultations to be conducted at home. This should include coverage for the doctor’s travel expenses to the patient's residence, as well as transportation costs for both the patient and their mobility technology, when traveling to specialized clinics for procedures such as ultrasounds, colonoscopies, medical rehabilitation, and other treatments aimed at restoring physical function or addressing disabilities.

In Romania, in 2024, I attempted to travel by wheelchair from my home, to the nearest ultrasound office. However, the clinic was located on the first floor of a building without an elevator, and the sidewalk was not accessible. As a result, I had to navigate the road unsafely. Upon arriving at the medical provider’s location, I found it impossible to go upstairs, even with the assistance of three accompanying adults, as they lacked a mobile elevator.

I was forced to call emergency services (112), and the rescue team carried me up the stairs in their arms. They had to remain on-site until I received my medical certificate. However, lifting the wheelchair upstairs presented significant difficulties. Mobility technologies are required to have safety belts, yet the 112 crew did not have a belt for wheelchair transport on stairs or a lifting belt for secure handling.

A bailiff assessed the situation and confirmed that the building’s infrastructure was inaccessible for my wheelchair, issuing an official report. Upon request, SMURD and 112 services provided me with a report detailing the assistance I received from the firefighters during my transport.

The three witnesses who accompanied me also provided a statement acknowledging their inability to assist due to a lack of necessary equipment, training, and expertise.

Despite multiple court rulings requiring the General Directorate of Social Assistance and Child Protection to provide live travel assistance and the necessary mobility technology, the agency failed to respond to any of my requests. Complaints of negligence and abuse filed against this entity were disregarded. Although the court overturned the initial decision by the prosecutor's office and ordered an investigation, no action was taken.

I also petitioned the court for an emergency order to ensure the safe transport of my wheelchair up the stairs, but was unsuccessful. Every legal effort failed—not only did I not receive the necessary ultrasound, but I was also unable to follow my doctor's medical recommendations, due to the lack of social and transport assistance.

As a result, my health deteriorated, and the only family member assisting me—who also has a disability—suffered further impairment. Instead of receiving the essential support to which I was entitled, my situation worsened, leading to additional hardship.

Social assistance services failed to provide adequate travel support.

Conclusions

Every medical or public institution should have adaptations for the wheelchair users and for any persons with mobility disorders.

The social workers need more education regarding the assisted mobility.

General Conclusions

Ioana Soare

This book gathers the experience of working 30 years in the assessment and 20 years in the legislation and theory in the insurance medicine. It promotes a few new ideas:

- a new definition for the insurance medicine;
- medico-social guidelines in the insurance medicine,
- comparisons of the social support and the life satisfaction among the disability onset groups;
- the independence of the physician/medical doctor working in insurance medicine, same as the accountant/auditor expert or the technical expert;
- a new psychological approach to the money we give to disabled people – not allowance, benefit, compensation, all having a discriminatory connotation, not pension which is for life, but simply money for health care; money for short/ long-term sick leave.

One can object that I emphasize the medical model of disability. Well, if I would have preferred the social model, that would have been discrimination, no?

The medical model may be widened to contain also some ideas of the handicapped role, is easily accepted by the patient and represents the first reason for asking for insurance rights.

Let us hope for a better collaboration between the state insurance companies/social protection systems and the private insurers, for a common language, in the years to come.

ANNEX

ORGANIZATIONS OF INSURANCE UNDERWRITERS

Abbr.	Region	Website	Association
AHOU	USA	www.ahou.org	Association of Home Office Underwriters
ELHUA	Europe	www.elhua.org	European Life and Health Underwriters' Association (2009)
LADUCA	New Zealand	www.laduca.co.nz	Association of Life And Disability Underwriting & Claims Assessors of New Zealand (2008)
AIU	India	http://aiu.experiencesense.com/	Association of Insurance Underwriters

https://www.iclam.org/insurance-medicine-links/

REGIONAL ORGANIZATIONS OF INSURANCE MEDICINE

NB: This list is focused on insurance medicine (private insurances), not on social security.

Abbr.	Region	Website	Association
AIMA	Asia	https://aima-org.com/en/index.html	AIMA Association
CEECLAM	Central-East Europe	http://www.ptmu.org.pl/en/	Central-Eastern European Committee for Life Disability and Health Assurance Medicine (2001)

NATIONAL ORGANIZATIONS OF INSURANCE MEDICINE

Abbr.	**Country**	**Website**	**Association**
ALUCA	Australasia	www.aluca.com	Australasian Life Underwriting and Claims Association (1986)
ACDMAV CLIMOA	Canada	www.climoa. com	Association Canadienne des Directeurs Médicaux en Assurance-Vie Canadian Life Insurance Medical Officers Association (1945)
FLF	Denmark	www.forsikrings laeger.dk	Forsikringslægernes Forening (1901)
SVY	Finland	www.vakuutusla kimiehet.fi	Suomen Vakuutuslääkärien Yhdistys
AMCAP	France	amcap.fr	Association des Médecins Conseils en Assurances de Personnes (1989)
DVFVW	Germany	www.dvfvw.de	Deutscher Verein für Versicherungswissenschaft e.V. (1899)
MEBOT	Hungary	www.mebot.hu	Magyar Életbiztosítási Orvostani Társaság
AIMAV	Italy	www.aimav.it	Associazione Italiana di Medicine dell'Assicurazione Vita, Malattia e Danni alla Persona (1959)
AIMJ	Japan	aimj.org	Association of Insurance Medicine of Japan (1901)
GAV	Netherlands	www.gav.nl	Nederlandse Vereniging van Geneeskundig Adviseurs in particuliere Verzekeringszaken (1901)

PAIM	Poland	www.ptmu.org.pl	Polskie Towarzystwo Medycyny Ubezpieczeniowej (1998)
ASISA AUCC	South-Africa	www.aucc.co.za	ASISA Underwriting & Claims Conference
AMES	Spain	www.amesred.com	Asociación Española del Medicina de Seguro
SIM	Switzerland	www.swiss-insurance-medicine.ch	Swiss Insurance Medicine (2003)
AMUS	United Kingdom	www.amus.org.uk	Assurance Medical & Underwriting Society (1893)
AAIM	USA	www.aaimedicine.org	American Academy of Insurance Medicine (1889)

CONTRIBUTORS

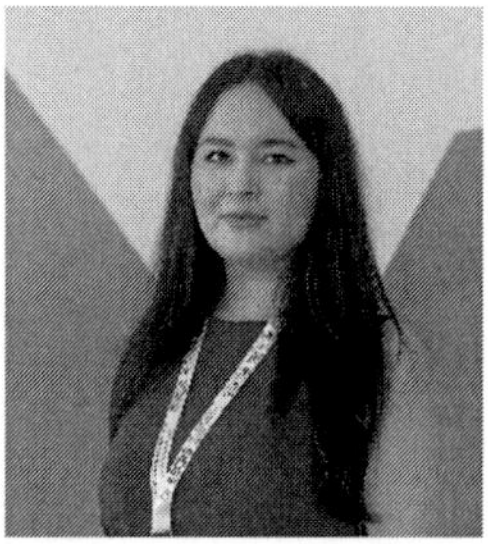

Suher ABDURAMAN, M.D.

Suher Abduraman was born on November 2, 1998. She graduated from the Faculty of Medicine at the "Ovidius" University of Constanța. She is a resident ophthalmologist at the Clinical Emergency Eye Hospital from Bucharest. She is specializing in the anterior pole pathology and the medical treatments of retina. Interested in technical novelties, Suher published several articles on the assistive devices and the computer programs for visually impaired people.

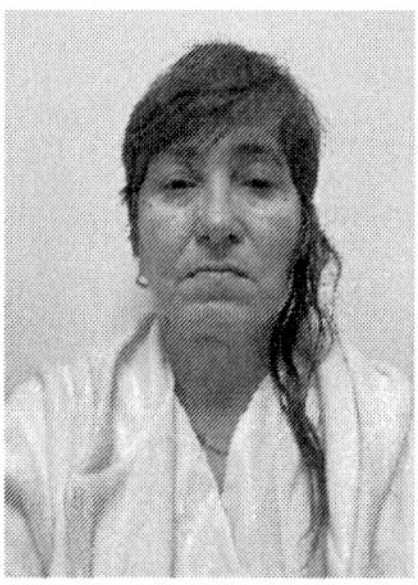

Laura BATIS, M.D., Ph.D. student

Dr. Batis works since 2000 as a m.d. in family medicine and geriatrics. Since 2023, she is an external collaborator at Titu Maiorescu University, Bucharest, Romania and since 2024 also a Ph.D. student. She held several positions as a medical manager in the last years.

Currently she works in the Department of Prehospital Emergencies at the Clinical Emergency Hospital Sf. Ioan, Bucharest, Romania.

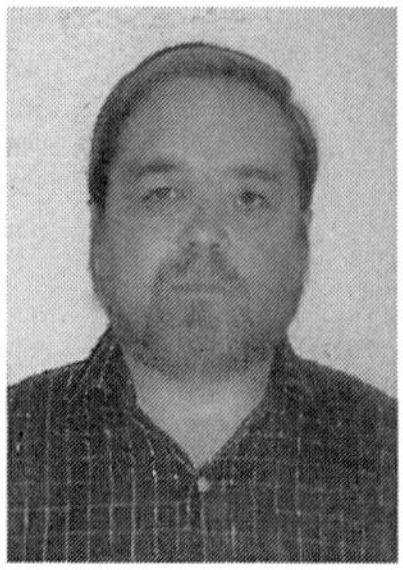

Valentin Eugen CIOCŞAN, M.D.

Born on November 3rd 1962 in Pucioasa, Dâmboviţa county, Romania. Graduated in 1988, Faculty of General Medicine Carol Davila University, Bucharest, Romania. Worked as a Family Physician in Pucioasa, Romania 1992-2007. He was a clinical coordinator in an American military base in Iraq 2007- 2008.

2009 -2016 he worked as a Disability Analyst at ATOS Healthcare/ Maximus, Coventry, UK. He is a fulltime poet and phantasy writer.

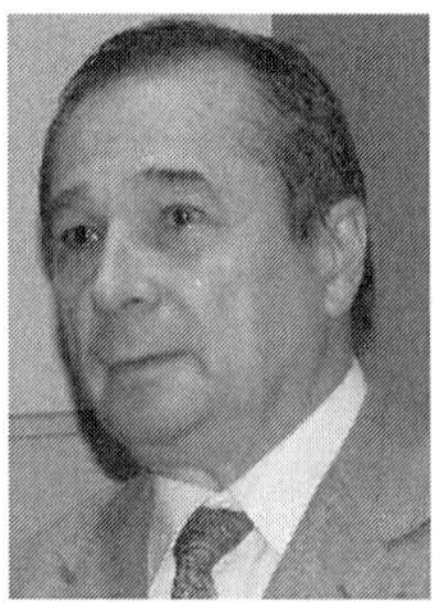

Manole COJOCARU, M.D., Ph.d.

Manole COJOCARU was born in 1951 in Bucharest, Romania. He graduated from the Faculty of Medicine, University of Medicine and Pharmacy Carol Davila, Bucharest, Romania, where he obtained MD title in 1977, and his PhD in 1997, and he is currently Research Scientist degree I (SciRes I). He is a specialist in laboratory medicine from 1984, and a specialist in allergology and clinical immunology from 1997. He is an

European specialist in laboratory medicine (EuSpLM). Since 2009 he is a Professor of Allergology and Clinical Immunology at Titu Maiorescu University, Faculty of Medicine, Bucharest. From 2023 he is an associate member of the Academy of Romanian Scientists. He has a remarkable publishing activity with more than 254 research items in peer-reviewed journals and several books. He has more than 3300 citations, h-index 27, i10-index 63. He has received several awards (Prize Lundbeck, Denmark, 2008; Prize EFNS, Helsinki, Finland, 2003; Roger Boeckx Memorial Award, Washington, USA, 2001).

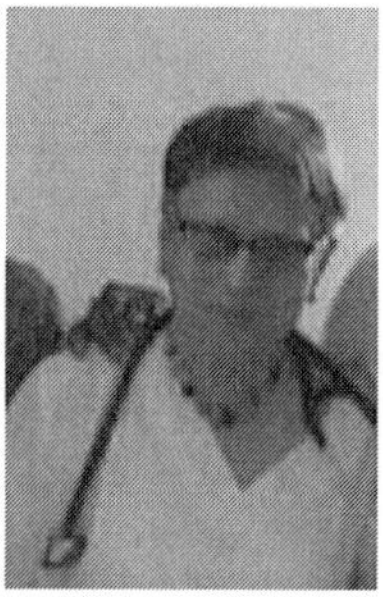

Gabriela Silvia GHEORGHE, M.D, Ph.D,

Dr. Gheorghe, cardiologist at Theodor Burghele Hospital Bucharest, Romania, was an assoc. prof. at Carol Davila University Bucharest, Romania. (1956-2024) Since 1993, she worked as an university assistant at UMF Carol Davila, at the Medical Clinic of the Caritas hospital, where she obtained her second specialty in cardiology and her doctorate. Since 2011, after the dissolution of the Caritas hospital, she worked at the Theodor Burghele Clinical Hospital, where she advanced to the position of associate professor in 2015. She worked in the Theodor Burghele hospital at the Cardiac Intensive Care Unit, where she selflessly cared for seriously ill patients, till her last days. She was in charge of the culture magazine Cugetarea Europeana where she produced the photo column and published very interesting articles. She was author of numerous books and articles, from which we mention ECG, from Theory to Practice, three editions at Etna Publishing House.

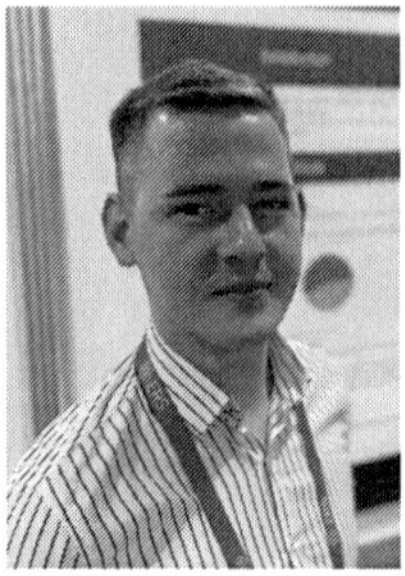

Constantin GHIMUȘ, MD, Ph.D. student in Pulmonary rehabilitation, Clinic of Pneumology, Clinical Hospital of Pneumophtisiology, Iassy, Romania

Constantin Ghimuş is a pulmonologist and PhD student in Pulmonary Rehabilitation under the supervision of Assoc. Prof. Habil. Dr. Paraschiva Postolache at the "Grigore T. Popa" University of Medicine and Pharmacy in Iaşi. With 5 years of residency training in pulmonology, Dr. Ghimuş combines clinical practice with academic and research activities.

In addition to his medical specialization, Dr. Ghimuş holds a nursing certification and a diploma in psycho-pedagogy, which enable him to approach patient care holistically, integrating educational and social aspects into his practice. He actively performs on-call duties in internal medicine and pulmonology departments.

Dr. Ghimuş is a volunteer with the Caritas organization, contributing to improving patient access to medical services. He has participated in numerous national and international congresses, presenting papers and engaging with renowned experts in the field of pulmonology. He has also authored scientific articles, reviews, and book chapters, thus enriching the medical literature.

His areas of interest include interstitial lung diseases, advanced patient monitoring technologies, the use of artificial intelligence in pulmonology, the management of chronic obstructive pulmonary diseases, and health education. Dr. Ghimuş is passionate about implementing innovations and lifelong learning, dedicating himself to enhancing the quality of medical care.

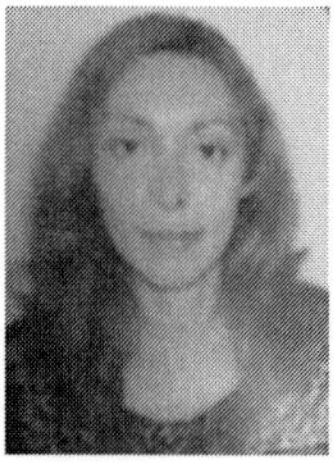

Roxana Elena MIRICA, M.D., Ph. D.

Lecturer in Insurance Medicine, at Carol Davila University Bucharest, Romania, where I train resident physicians in the social insurance medicine field, highlighting the steps that a patient should follow to retire due to illness, according to current legislation.

I graduated from the Faculty of Medicine in 2000, since 2006 I have been working both at the Carol Davila University of Medicine and Pharmacy in Bucharest and at the National Institute of Medical Expertise and Work Capacity Recovery. I sustained my doctoral thesis in 2009.

Also, I am a Gastroenterologist, specialized in abdominal ultrasound, working at Regina Maria, Private Healthcare Network, Bucharest, Romania.

In my capacity as an academic, I have published medical articles in both national and international specialized journals (9 articles in international medical journals, about 30 articles in national medical journals and 1 international book chapter).

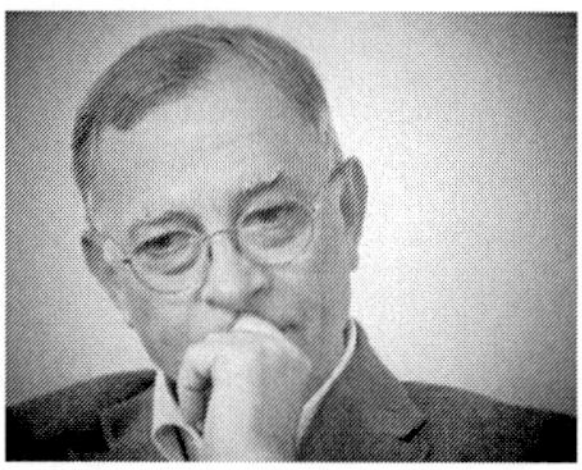

Alexandru-Eugen NICOLAU, M.D., Ph. D., (1953-2024)

Dr. Nicolau graduated from UMF "Iuliu Hatieganu" Cluj-Napoca in 1978 and became doctor of medical sciences since 2001.

He had skills of laparoscopic surgery and medical management. He completed classic and laparoscopic surgery internships in prestigious services in Belgium and Switzerland.

He worked at the Clinic of Surgery, Clinical Hospital of Emergency, Bucharest, Romania 1981-2023, where he performed the first laparoscopic operations in Dec. 1993, the first in this hospital and among the first in Romania.

He was the author of more than 50 scientific articles published in domestic and foreign magazines, and he contributed to 12 surgical manuals and books, including the original monograph "Emergency laparoscopic surgery".

He was in the board of ARCE (Romanian Association of Endoscopic Surgery) and in the board of the Abdominal trauma section of ESTES (European Association for Trauma and Emergency Surgery).

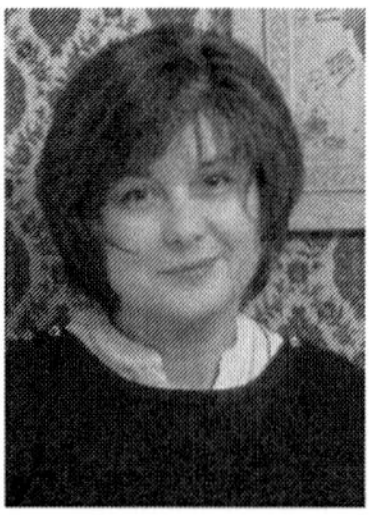

Anca PAVEL, M.D., Ph.d, occupational medicine, France

Graduated from UMF Carol Davila, Bucharest in 1988. From 1994 is a specialist physician in occupational medicine and obtained her PhD in 2001. She worked as a university assistant at UMF Carol Davila, 1991-2000 and in the same period at Colentina Hospital, Occupational Diseases clinic.

Dr. Anca Pavel worked as an assoc. prof. at Titu Maiorescu University 2000-2012 and in the same period had clinical integration at Witting hospital, internal medicine clinic. She was vice dean to the Faculty of Medicine at Titu Maiorescu University.

Since 2012 she works as an Occupational medicine physician at SPSTI 81 (Service paritaire en santé au travail interentreprises du Tarn), Albi, France.

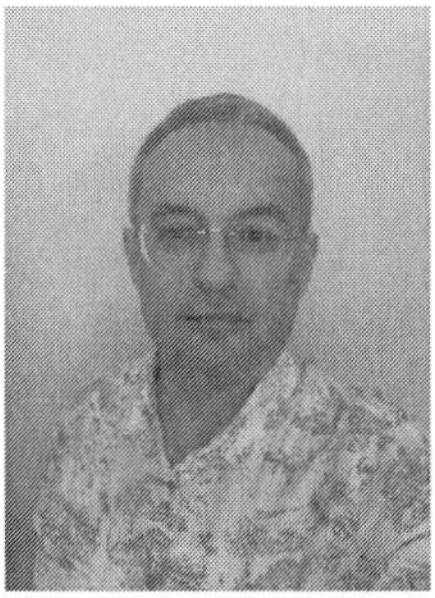

Nicolae PAUN, M.D., Ph.D.

Born on the 1st of May 1966, dr. Paun graduated from the Faculty of Medicine, Carol Davila University of Medicine and Pharmacy, Bucharest, Romania as MD in 1990 and sustained his PhD in Medical sciences in 2006.

He currently holds the position of associated professor at the Carol Davila University of Medicine and Pharmacy, department of Cardiology. He is a Senior Cardiologist at the Prof. Dr. Theodor Burghele Hospital, Bucharest. He has authored many articles and published in important journals of Cardiology and Internal Medicine. He was the main author in observational studies in echocardiography, rewarded with Ist prize at the National Congresses of Echocardiography.

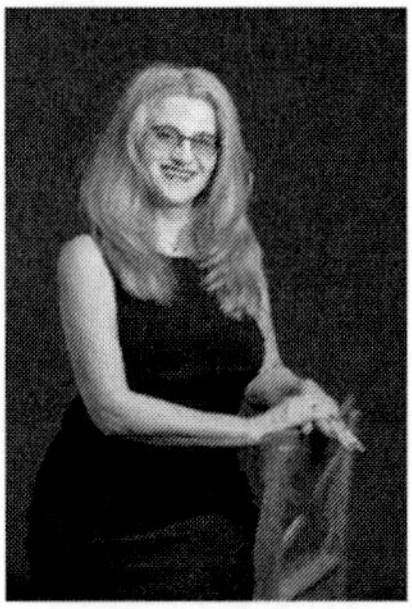

Paraschiva A. POSTOLACHE MD, PhD, FCCP, Prof. Habil. "Grigore T. Popa" University of Medicine and Pharmacy, Iași, Romania, Faculty of Medicine, Department of Medical Sciences I; Rehabilitation Clinical Hospital, Iași, Romania - Head of the Respiratory Rehabilitation Clinic.

Prof. Habil. Dr. Paraschiva POSTOLACHE is a faculty member at the "Grigore T. Popa" University of Medicine and Pharmacy in Iași, Faculty of Medicine, Department of Medical Sciences I, and the Faculty of Medical Bioengineering. She is a physician specialized in: Internal Medicine, Pulmonology, Clinical Pharmacology and an international specialist in Rehabilitation and Physical Medicine. She is also certified as Smoking Cessation Counselor. Paraschiva Postolache serves as the Coordinator of the Smoking Cessation Counselling Centre at the Rehabilitation Clinical Hospital in Iassy and Member of the National Smoking Cessation Program "STOP SMOKING" of the Romanian Ministry of Health. She is a National Expert in Clinical Pharmacology and Toxicology, as well as a European Expert in Disability and Rehabilitation of the Romanian Ministry of Health. Within the Romanian Society of Pulmonology (RSP), Paraschiva Postolache is the Founder (2006) and Coordinator of the Respiratory Rehabilitation Working Group and member of the RSP Board of Directors (2012–2020; 2022–present).

Prof. Paraschiva Postolache has an extensive scientific, educational, and editorial activity, both nationally and internationally, in the field of respiratory rehabilitation. She is recognized as the initiator, organizer, and developer of this domain in Romania. Prof. Paraschiva POSTOLACHE is acknowledged as an expert and leader in respiratory rehabilitation, with over 1,000 invited lectures and more than 250 full-text publications in national and international journals, as well as books and book chapters published by national and international publishers. Her contributions include reviews, peer reviews, national and international projects and grants coordination, and membership in editorial boards of international and national journals.

Prof. Paraschiva Postolache has represented Romania at CHEST / American College of Chest Physicians (ACCP) as a Member of the Board of Regents, Chair of the CHEST Council of Global Governors, and Member of the CHEST Council of Regents (2011–2014). She has also served as a Member of the Steering Committee for the Pulmonary Physiology, Function, and Rehabilitation Network of CHEST/ACCP (2014–2018) and has been a Member of the CHEST Council of Global Governors since 2011. Dr. Postolache has been a CHEST/ACCP Regent and Global Governor for Romania since 2006, an ACCP Fellow (FCCP), USA, since 2005, and a National GOLD Leader for Romania, 2010, for the European Respiratory Society.

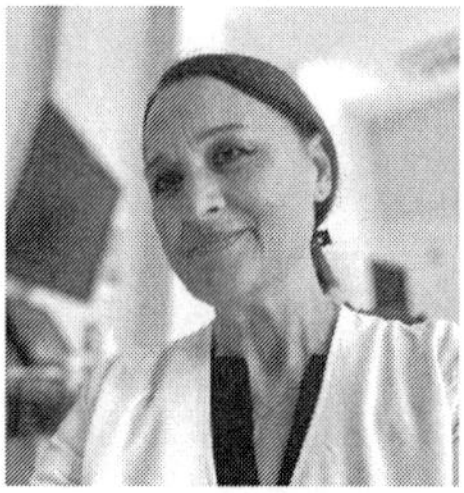

Camer SALIM, M.D., Ph. D., Assoc.Prof. in Emergency Medicine, Faculty of Medicine, "Ovidius" University of Constanța

Dr. Camer Salim, born on April 30, 1966, in Constanța, Romania, graduated from the University of Medicine and Pharmacy, Târgu Mureș, în 1991, with top honors (GPA: 10). She earned her **Ph.D. in Medicine** in 2004, focusing on the microscopic diagnosis of neuroendocrine tumors. Over her 30-year career, Dr. Camer has combined clinical excellence with academic contributions. She serves as a Physician in Emergency Medicine at the Constanța County Emergency Clinical Hospital (SCJU) and as an Endocrinology Consultant at CARDIOMEDSAL, Constanța. Additionally, she has held key administrative roles, including Medical Director and President of the Ethics Committee at Constanța Clinical Emergency Hospital.

As a former Assistant Professor at the Faculty of Medicine, University "Ovidius" Constanța, dr. Camer taught Anatomy and contributed to shaping future medical professionals. She has authored several books and peer-reviewed articles, including a Practical Guide for Cardiovascular Emergencies in Dentistry and studies on the brain-gut axis in Parkinson's disease management and neuroanatomy of cerebellum.

Fluent in English, French, Turkish, and Tatar, she is a proponent of interdisciplinary collaboration in advancing patient care and medical education.

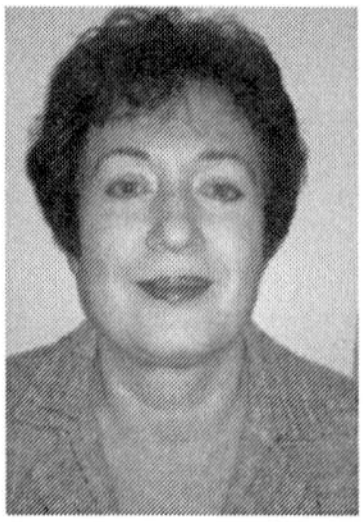

Ioana SOARE, M.D., Ph. D., lecturer in Insurance Medicine, University Titu Maiorescu, Bucharest, Romania

Ioana Soare was born in 1963 in Bucharest, Romania. She graduated from the Faculty of Medicine, Carol Davila University of Medicine and Pharmacy, Bucharest, Romania, where she obtained MD title in 1988 and her Ph.D. in 2006. Since 2010 she is a lecturer at Titu Maiorescu University, Faculty of Medicine and Faculty of Nursing.

Member of the Medical Expertise Commission of the Romanian College of Physicians, from 2007 until 2020.

Member of the General Council of EUMASS, 2009-2019, the European association of insurance expert doctors.

Member of the Bureau of ICLAM, the World association of medical insurance experts, since 2012.

Current president of the Professional Association Corpul Medicilor Experti de Asigurari, CMEA, Health and Life Insurance Medical Experts since 2015.

Member in the Council of PERGAM, the association of scientific writings authors.

Medical expert in court since 2005, in over 100 different cases in road and work accidents.

Author of 8 handbooks and medical books, including Insurance Medicine, 2010 and Medical expertise, Insurance Medicine Handbook, 2017.

Author of over 100 scientific articles and chapters on medical expertise, in Romania, in the USA.

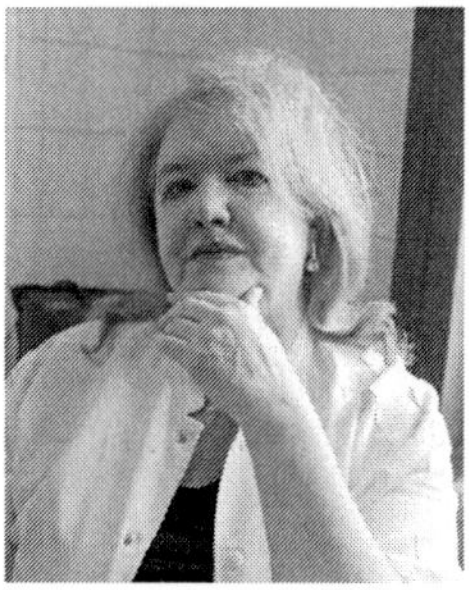

Simona Liana SOARE, M.D., Ph. D., lecturer in Internal Medicine, University Titu Maiorescu, Bucharest, Romania

Born in 1955, Simona Liana Soare graduated from the Faculty of Medicine, Carol Davila University of Medicine and Pharmacy, Bucharest, Romania, where she obtained MD title in 1980 and her PhD in 2000. Since 2014 she is a lecturer at Titu Maiorescu University, Faculty of Medicine. She is a physician specialized in Internal Medicine and Rheumatology, working at the Elias Emergency University Hospital, Bucharest, Romania. Author of medical books and many scientific articles, she is member of Romanian Society of Rheumatology, Romanian Society of Internal Medicine.

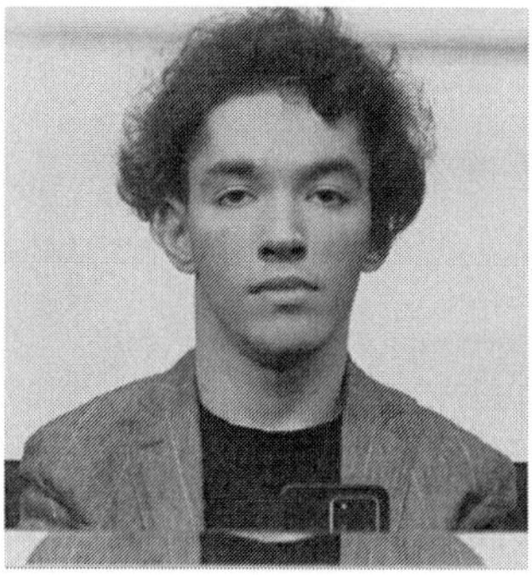

Ștefan Moshe STOIAN, lawyer

I am a law graduate and the only A in my series of master in business law. Being a law professional and a person with mobility issues, I became an independent expert of the Monitoring Council of the implementation of the Convention on the Rights of Persons with Disabilities, adopted in New York by the United Nations General Assembly on December 13, 2006, signed by Romania on September 26, 2007 and ratified by Romania through law

221/2010. In order to ensure a punctual access, we established the Facebook page "Coalitia nedeplasabilului" https://www.facebook.com/groups/779799468763551 for people with the same type of disability, in order to identify a solution as uniform as possible.

I have intervened in many legislative changes, I have filed over 9000 criminal complaints and I have about 130 active civil cases pending today and countless non-discrimination petitions. I like to help and I breathe for a better world in which I have a place too. I strongly believe that for any problem there is a solution and I am living proof that despite the disability, there is success.

I am campaigning for the rights of people with disabilities and for the helpless, but also for the creation of opportunities for them, of access to legal services, to the physical environment and to the law in order to equalize opportunities.

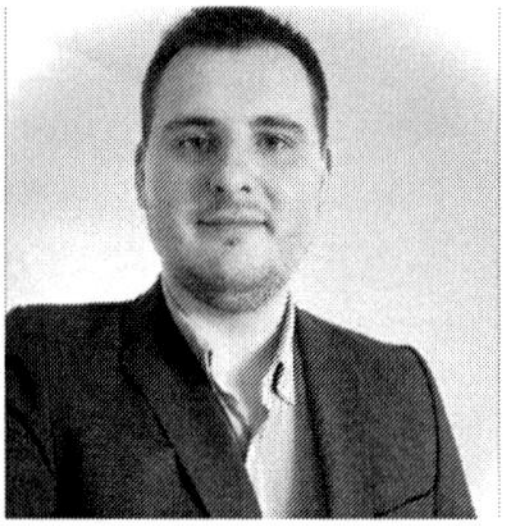

Ştefan Săndulache, M.D., Department I Pneumology, Clinical Hospital of Pneumophthisiology, Iasi, Romania

Ştefan Săndulache is a physician specialized in Pulmonology working at the Clinical Hospital of Pneumophthisiology, Iasi (Romania). After 5 years of residency training, his areas of interest are the diagnosis and treatment of interstitial lung diseases (idiopathic pulmonary fibrosis, hypersensitivity pneumonitis, sarcoidosis, interstitial lung diseases secondary to collagen diseases such as rheumatoid arthritis or systemic scleroderma), somnology and pulmonary rehabilitation (which is the basis of non-pharmacological treatment of patients with chronic lung diseases and more). He actively performs on-call duties in the pulmonology departments.

Dr. Săndulache has participated in numerous courses and congresses, both national and international, presenting papers and collaborating with renowned experts in the field of respiratory medicine. He is also the author of scientific articles and book chapters, thus enriching the specialized literature. Since medical school, Dr. Săndulache has been a writer and editor for 4 years of a website of medical articles in his country, precisely out of the desire to bring accurate medical information as close as possible to patients and healthy people.

In addition to his current medical activity in the hospital, Dr. Săndulache is an associate professor at the Post-Secondary High School of Health Sciences "Prof. Dr. P. Branzei" Iasi, training future nurses in the field of the internal medicine and the medical emergencies.